VIRUS
GROUND ZERO

Also by Ed Regis

Nano
Great Mambo Chicken and the Transhuman Condition
Who Got Einstein's Office?

VIRUS
GROUND ZERO

Stalking the Killer Viruses with the Centers for Disease Control

Ed Regis

POCKET BOOKS
New York   London   Toronto   Sydney   Tokyo   Singapore

POCKET BOOKS, a division of Simon & Schuster Inc.
1230 Avenue of the Americas, New York, NY 10020

ISBN: 0-671-55361-5

First Pocket Books hardcover printing November 1996

10 9 8 7 6 5 4 3 2 1

For
Jean V. Naggar

Contents

VIRUS
GROUND ZERO

Prologue: A Mother and Daughter

It was quiet in there. It was so very quiet that she heard nothing at all for long stretches of time, nothing but the breathing sounds of her mother, her very own mother, who was lying in bed with her, lying in the same hospital bed in which Loki M'Bele now lay. Loki M'Bele was twenty years old, her mother was forty-two, and they were the only two living souls in the small, quiet room. It had been the measles ward, children once lay in those beds, but there were no longer any children here. In fact, only one other person was in the measles ward, a patient in the bed across the aisle.

An IV bottle hung from a hook above the patient's head, and a tube ran down from the bottle to a needle stuck in his arm. An intravenous solution had been dripping into his arm, but now the IV bottle was empty and dry. He had lain there like that, in his own dried blood and bodily effusions, his bloodshot eyes staring up at the ceiling, for the last couple of days. The patient was dead.

1

In the afternoon, some men came into the room from the outside. They looked around but said nothing, and they did not touch the patients. Then they were gone.

Loki M'Bele's mother was breathing very fast now, making short, quick gulping noises, gasping for air, trying to force a single good breath into her lungs.

Later that night, her mother, still lying next to her in the same bed, stopped breathing.

The next day, the men came again. They wore face masks and surgical caps and ankle-length gowns, and they lifted Loki M'Bele up off the bed, placed her on a moving cart, and wheeled the cart out of the measles ward. They wheeled her out into the open air, across the grass courtyard, and onto a covered walkway.

A distance from the covered walkway, on the outside face of a concrete wall, a sign said:

RÉPUBLIQUE DU ZAIRE
RÉGION DE BANDUNDU
VILLE DE KIKWIT
Hôpital Général

Kikwit General Hospital had 326 beds distributed out in ten separate buildings called pavilions. The pavilions had no electricity, no running water, and no proper sanitation. There was no bathroom and no kitchen, and the hospital provided no meals to its patients.

The moving cart squeaked as it went. Some goats were lying down on the covered walkway and they got up as the cart moved past.

The men wheeled Loki M'Bele into Pavilion 3. Pavilion 3 contained a long, open ward room with sixteen beds, eight on either side of a center aisle. The hospital attendants wheeled

Loki M'Bele down the center aisle, lifted her up off the cart, and placed her in one of the empty beds.

She lay on her back on a thin mattress without sheets, on a metal bedframe whose faded white paint had chipped off and worn away over years of use. A rumpled, bright-colored blanket half-covered her body. Other patients were in the ward room, on other beds, and on the floor, and the whole room smelled of bleach. As she lay there now, she herself started to gulp for air in small, quick gasps. Her eyes opened wide in an expression of fright, as if she were about to scream. Then she vomited onto the mattress and the floor.

She lay there like that for the rest of the day. Through an open window above her head she could see the lower surface of the overhanging roof. The sun was setting behind the trees, shining in through the open doorway at the far end of the room, the light slanting in with an orange tint.

Now it was evening, almost night. A kerosene lantern sat on a table, but it had not been lit, and so it was quite dark in the pavilion. The beds, the patients, and the blue walls were fading from view, becoming soft and imprecise.

Then Loki M'Bele could hear voices from the outside, the sounds of people talking. And then the voices were coming closer, a couple of people.

She could hear footsteps, the squish of rubber boots on wet concrete, and she could see flashlight beams: spots of light bobbing up and down on the walls and along the floor.

Then, two figures were inside the pavilion. They moved among the beds, stopping for a moment at the different patients. One of the figures had a miner's lamp strapped to his head, and it lit up his gloved hands as he washed a patient's skin with a cloth.

After a while one of the figures came toward Loki M'Bele.

"How do you feel?" he asked in French.

Loki M'Bele gasped for air.

He felt her pulse.

3

Finally she said, "Water . . . please . . . juice."

A plastic water bottle sat on the table across the room. The figure walked to it, poured out some water into a cup, and brought it to Loki M'Bele. She did not extend her hand for the cup, so he reached down and supported her head, and she took a few sips.

Then the figure moved away, the flashlight glare now out of her eyes. She saw that both of the men were leaving, moving back out of the pavilion. She saw the spots of light bobbing to and fro around the room. They were the last things she saw.

Next morning her body was sprayed with bleach, placed in a white plastic bag, and sprayed again. Then it was put on a gurney and wheeled to the morgue.

The morgue was some distance from Pavilion 3, down the covered walkway and back out across the grass. The small concrete building had a single door, a door that was always open now, because there'd been so many deaths at Kikwit General Hospital. A line of other bleach-sprayed bodies covered the floor of the morgue, and the attendants placed the body of Loki M'Bele next to them.

It was not the ideal place for any sort of postmortem procedure, much less for a formal autopsy: there were no stainless steel examination tables here, no floodlights, no automated scales with digital readouts giving you the precise weight of each of the body's various organs as you placed them in the hopper. There was just a concrete floor, oozing and slippery with blood, bodily secretions, and sprayed bleach.

But a tissue sample would prove beyond doubt what it was that Loki M'Bele had died from, and so one of the figures from the night before—masked and gowned, wearing a cap, goggles, and a clean white surgical apron—now crouched over the body bag.

He opened up the body bag. He pushed back a layer of

clothing, revealing Loki M'Bele's dark skin. He swabbed the skin with alcohol, and then carefully, deliberately, making sure that the sharp edge of the knife pointed away from himself at all times, he made an incision into the abdomen just above the navel. He pulled back the skin flaps, made another incision, and found the liver. He shoved a biopsy needle into the liver, twisted it, and pulled it out again.

He turned and dropped the sample into a plastic vial, which he placed into a box. He closed the body bag. He picked up his scalpel and sample box, stood up, and took a last look around.

Then he got out of there.

1   The Call

Word of the Kikwit outbreak reached the Centers for Disease Control at 4:20 in the afternoon of Saturday, May 6, 1995. Unfortunately, on Saturdays the CDC was closed. So instead of going into the main switchboard, the call came into the reception desk in the lobby of the administration building where it was answered by Diane Hairston-Nash, a security guard who worked there nights and weekends.

The caller was not, as might be expected, a harried doctor at the Kikwit hospital. Nor was it a Zairian public-health official. The caller was one Julia Weeks, an American physician at a private nonprofit clinic in Zaire, who at that moment was speaking into her personal cellular telephone while sitting on a bench overlooking the tennis courts at the British embassy in Kinshasa.

"I think we've got an outbreak of Ebola virus down here," she said over the phone. "I'd like to talk to somebody about it."

She'd learned about the epidemic just that very morning.

She'd been at work at the Zaire-American Clinic, of which she was the medical director, when a friend of hers, Larry Streshley, who did public health work for the Presbyterian mission in Kinshasa, stopped in for a piece of advice. He'd been in radio contact with a hospital in the interior of the country, in Kikwit, where there was this huge outbreak of red diarrhea, also known as shigella.

"He was getting a bunch of stuff together to send on a plane that was to go from Kinshasa to Kikwit," Julia Weeks recalled later. "He was getting together drugs to deal with it, and we were discussing which antibiotics would be most appropriate, and which were available, and what sort of equipment they would need, in terms of gloves and gowns, to help provide some barrier care."

This in itself was not unusual: shigella was common enough all throughout Africa. So she made a few suggestions and Larry Streshley left. That night, she attended a cocktail party at the British embassy. Many of the guests were talking about the new outbreak, but now a rumor was going around that it was not in fact shigella, but rather Ebola, a viral hemorrhagic fever with a fatality rate of up to 90 percent. Some of the guests came up to Julia Weeks and asked her about it.

"As far as I've heard, from the symptoms that were presented to me this morning, it wouldn't be Ebola," she told them.

But then Gerald Scott, the American DCM—the deputy chief of mission—introduced her to Dan Pader, an official of the Catholic Church in Zaire, who was also at the party. Pader had just talked with some nuns who'd actually been at the hospital in Kikwit and who had a more precise description of the symptoms. The initial symptoms were fever and bloody diarrhea, that was true. But then within a few days there was this massive bleeding from all over, blood pouring out of all the body's pores and other openings: mouth, nose, everywhere else. Finally the victims lost consciousness, after which they literally bled to death.

Oh, my God, Julia Weeks thought to herself. *Shigella doesn't do that. This is not shigella, this is a hemorrhagic fever, absolutely. Just like what they described as Ebola in 1976.*

"Look, this is serious," she told the American deputy. "The only people who are going to know what to do about this are the CDC. We really should call the CDC."

Which she was doing right now from the embassy backyard, away from the other guests, three diplomats standing next to her, cocktail glasses in hand, people from the party glancing her way across the lawn, talking amongst themselves while looking in her direction as she looked back at them and waited for someone from the CDC to come back on the line.

"Hello, this is Ali Khan," a voice said.

Ali Khan was a thirty-one-year-old CDC physician and epidemiologist who was at that point putting in some quality time at home with his wife and the triplets. He was not related to Aly Khan, the playboy, or to the Aga Khan, the playboy's multimillionaire father, or to Genghis Khan or to any of the other famous Khans, but he somewhat resembled the actor Omar Sharif. He was dark-skinned and wore a mustache, and although he grew up mostly in Pakistan, Ali Khan had been born in Brooklyn and spoke with no trace of an accent. He was extremely businesslike and precise in manner, and totally committed to the theory and practice of public health. He was also one of only five people on the CDC's in-house list of whom to call when the reported problem was Ebola.

So Julia Weeks now told Ali Khan the whole story: one or two thousand people either sick, dead, or dying. Fever, bloody diarrhea, blood oozing from intravenous sites, uncontrollable bleeding, the victims essentially hemorrhaging to death. No response to Cipro, Bactrim, or any other antibiotic that had been administered. Twelve members of a surgical team—doctors, nurses, assistants—had died.

"It was a very scary story," Ali Khan recalled later.

It was scary because, for one thing, the symptoms did indeed bear all the earmarks of a viral hemorrhagic fever. It was probably not shigella, whose major symptom was also bloody diarrhea, because shigella responded well to antibiotics, which this condition wasn't doing. It might be yellow fever, just possibly, but the doctors and nurses who'd died had probably been vaccinated against yellow fever, so chances were good it wasn't that.

Which left, among other things, Marburg and Ebola, which ranked among the most frightening diseases of all time. They appeared out of nowhere, there was no treatment for them— no drugs, vaccines, no therapies of any sort. They were beyond the reach of medical science: the victims just got sick, bled away, and died.

The worst part of it was, those diseases had a track record of being highly transmissible by direct contact, especially in rural, poorly equipped hospitals, which this site in Kikwit gave every indication of being. In such settings, the viruses went from one person to the next by touch, and if unchecked, they were capable of spreading out in successive waves with amazing speed and lethal force.

The two doctors talked for about half an hour, at which point the batteries of Julia Weeks's cellular phone were beginning to give out. It was then 9:50 P.M. in Kinshasa and 4:50 P.M. in Atlanta. Ali Khan said he'd get in touch with some of the other people in the Special Pathogens Branch, where he worked, who'd doubtless want to talk to her themselves. Weeks said that she lived in the Chevron Oil Company compound, which had a reliable satellite phone system—one of the few dependable ways of making a call into or out of Zaire—so it would be best, she said, if they called her at home.

Ali hung up, said good-bye to Kristin and the kids—Rabi, Aliya, and Salim—and left for the office, a windowless, Spartan cubicle in the basement of Building 3. He got his boss on the phone, Clarence James Peters, M.D.

C. J. Peters was without a doubt the world's most glamorous living virologist. He was one of the heroes of Richard Preston's book *The Hot Zone*, which portrayed him, correctly, as the mastermind of the Reston biohazard operation, an effort in which he'd directed the euthanasia and disposal of 450 monkeys, many of them carrying the Ebola virus, in Reston, Virginia, an elegant wooded suburb of Washington, D.C. One of the more disturbing aspects of that outbreak was the way in which that particular strain of the virus—called Ebola Reston—had traveled from monkey to monkey through the air. There, at least, direct contact was not required for transmission: the virus could be, and had been, borne along on tiny aerosolized particles that floated here and there around the room, and from room to room within the building. Fortunately, Ebola Reston was not lethal to human beings, but if it had been . . . well, the prospect did not bear thinking about.

At the time of the Reston episode, Peters was chief of the disease assessment division of the United States Army Medical Research Institute of Infectious Diseases (USAMRIID), at Fort Detrick, Maryland. In the world of infectious-disease research and containment, only one position was higher up than that in terms of prestige, visibility, and ultimate responsibility: head of the Special Pathogens Branch at the CDC. When that position came open in 1992, C. J. Peters left for Atlanta.

By six o'clock that evening, Peters, Ali Khan, and Tom Ksiazek, the CDC's top lab man, were together in Khan's office working out a plan of action. Item one was to get hold of the specimens. Supposedly, blood samples had been taken from some of the Kikwit patients and put on a plane bound out of Zaire. Exactly where they were now, however, no one seemed to know for sure.

Item two was to fax Kinshasa with lists of instructions for diagnosing viral hemorrhagic fevers, for isolating patients, shipping additional specimens, and so forth.

Item three was to inform the higher-ups within the CDC—Brian Mahy and Jim Hughes—about the outbreak.

And then they were on the phone again with Julia Weeks.

Although Peters, Khan, and Ksiazek were intent on getting the blood samples that had been taken from the Kikwit patients, the specimens had not been addressed to, and had not been intended for, the Centers for Disease Control. They'd been meant for the Institute of Tropical Medicine in Antwerp, Belgium, which was where they were in fact headed.

A military nurse had drawn the blood from fourteen patients on May 4 and 5, at the suggestion of Tamfum Muyembe, the University of Kinshasa virologist who had been called in to assess the situation. Muyembe, a compact, rather boyish-looking Zairian, was an old hand at dealing with Ebola. He'd been at the original Ebola outbreak in the town of Yambuku, also in Zaire, back in 1976, and was all too familiar with what a developing epidemic of the disease looked like.

Muyembe had arrived in Kikwit from Kinshasa on May 1, had acquainted himself with the known history of the new outbreak, and had made a chart showing the lines of transmission among those who had died. From all this he'd concluded that a viral hemorrhagic fever of some sort was racing through Kikwit General Hospital.

The only way to know for sure was to send blood samples to a qualified lab, which would isolate the pathogen and positively identify it. There were no such labs in Zaire, however, and the lab that Muyembe had in mind was run by Guido van der Groen, a Belgian virologist at the Institute of Tropical Medicine in Antwerp. Zaire was formerly the Belgian Congo, and although the country had been independent since 1960, it had retained close ties to its mother country, which seemed to have a strong sense of obligation toward its former colony. There was still a large Belgian presence in Zaire, including an organization called the Belgian Development Cooperation, which provided medical aid to the country, among other things. So when Tamfum Muyembe packed and boxed the blood samples, he addressed them to Guido van der Groen at the Institute of Tropical Medicine. The one thing Muyembe didn't know was that the ITM no longer had the requisite biosafety lab and would not be able to process the samples.

Muyembe placed the samples in a metal canister, stuffed cotton wadding around each of the tubes, put the canister in a plastic box and then filled it with ice. He sealed it up and gave it to Monsignor Nicol, the French deputy bishop of Kikwit, along with a letter that Muyembe had typed out the day before, addressing it to Dr. Jean-Pierre Lahaye at the Belgian embassy in Kinshasa. He also enclosed his schematic diagram of the outbreak, *"Filiation des cas à Kikwit"* (Relationship among cases at Kikwit), showing the probable lines of transmission from victim to victim.

On Friday, May 5, Monsignor Nicol, together with another Kikwit priest, Father Richard P. Stark, left Kikwit aboard a Mission Air Fellowship single-engine Cessna flown by Fellowship pilot Tom Howard.

Monsignor Nicol delivered the samples to Dr. Lahaye in Kinshasa at 5 P.M. that same afternoon. Lahaye, who was in charge of the embassy's medical section, read Muyembe's cover letter, which asked him to open the box, renew the ice, and forward the specimens to Belgium.

The embassy's medical section was off in its own little annex attached to one side of the building. There was a biohazard freezer and a workbench in a separate room, so Lahaye went in there and opened the box, which was roughly the size and shape of a picnic cooler. He saw that the samples were still intact, added in some fresh ice, and sealed it all back up again.

The hard part would be getting the box out of Kinshasa and into Belgium. Doing everything by the book and through official channels, with all the rules and regulations being followed, the permissions, authorizations, and approvals being obtained from all the various and assorted bureaucrats, well, that could take forever, especially on a Friday night with the weekend coming up, and especially when what you were sending to Europe was not some innocuous little medical specimen but rather a tidy parcel of Marburg or Ebola or some other such thing.

That left the unofficial route. A Sabena flight was leaving Kinshasa at 9:25 P.M. local time, due to arrive in Brussels at 5:55 the following morning. And there was Claudia.

Claudia was a Sabena employee known to the embassy, a reliable Zairian woman who made frequent business trips between Kinshasa and Brussels. In fact she was scheduled to go out on the flight tonight. Supposing she'd cooperate, that would get the samples out of the country. But then there was the separate problem of getting them into Belgium, which was to say, getting them past the customs and immigration officials at Zaventem, the Brussels airport, who could not be expected to look favorably upon the whole arrangement. Lahaye had the Belgian ambassador in Kinshasa, André Moens, write a note on embassy letterhead explaining the situation, saying that the samples were not to be opened by anybody other than the doctors at the Institute of Tropical Medicine, and requesting that Claudia be allowed to pass through customs with the box in hand.

Claudia agreed to carry the samples, and so on Friday, May 5, about twelve hours before Julia Weeks ever heard the first thing about a possible outbreak of shigella in the backcountry, Claudia walked up the stairway to Sabena flight 556, bringing the sample box aboard as hand luggage. And as the plane, a Boeing 747, taxied out to the airport's three-mile-long runway, fourteen plastic tubes laden with one of the hottest viral agents known to humanity were riding along in a picnic cooler placed on the floor of the passenger cabin.

*   *   *

Two days later, with the location of the blood samples still unknown, C. J. Peters decided to send a medical team into Zaire. Peters was at that point fifty-five years old, slightly squat, with a cherubic, somewhat chipmunklike face. He sported a thin, gray mustache and smiled a lot and liked to laugh with this high-pitched yelp of his, and he was quick to see the humor, if any, in a given situation.

Not that there was much humor in the events currently unfolding around him. He'd been dealing with hemorrhagic fevers for much of his life and knew exactly how lethal they were. Long before the Ebola Reston outbreak, Peters had been in South America on the track of Bolivian hemorrhagic fever, also known as Machupo, when a friend of his who was doing an autopsy on a woman who'd died of the ailment let his knife slip. His friend was dead before the week was out.

So this was no business for amateurs. In fact, from Peters' point of view, it was the absolute worst type of epidemic, occurring thousands of miles away in a remote corner of a country, Zaire, that had poor diplomatic relations with the United States, no reliable telephone service, backward medical institutions, and not much in the way of sanitation, drugs, or barrier-nursing supplies. Those were conditions that promoted the rapid spread of a contagious disease. Anyone from the CDC who went over there would be exposing himself not only to the pathogen that was causing the outbreak but also to all the other diseases that were rife in Central Africa, which made up a long list of human afflictions. There was malaria, yellow fever, cholera, typhus, yaws, sleeping sickness, and so on and so forth. There seemed to be no end to the microbes you could encounter over there.

It was obvious that some outside help was needed because if the Zairian health authorities were equal to the task of containing the epidemic, then there would already have been some sign, however slight, that the outbreak was coming under control. Every report he received, however, gave him the precise opposite impression: the deaths were continuing, the disease was spreading, and nobody had the equipment, medicine, or know-how to stop it.

On Sunday, the day after he talked with Julia Weeks, C. J. Peters had a pretty good idea as to who from the CDC would be going into Zaire. Although there were innumerable dialects spoken by members of the more than two hundred Bantu and other ethnic groups in the country, French was the official language and widely understood, so Peters had in mind Pierre Rollin and Philippe Calain, two native French-speaking clinicians, plus Ali Khan, his top epidemiologist. The plan was that these three would travel to Kinshasa with a load of protective gear, stay overnight, then fly out to Kikwit the next morning and begin work. That work would center upon two things: interrupting the chain of transmission and tracing it back to its starting point.

Peters himself, unfortunately, would not be taking the trip because, for one thing, he spoke no French. Second, despite his having outwitted a large variety of the world's germs, he was at that point running a fever, coughing up some green goo, and was in no shape to lead any sort of field operation into the wilds of Africa. It would be enough if he'd be able to get it all rolling.

Step one of which was getting a request for help from the government of Zaire. The CDC could not simply barge into a country and start practicing medicine; it couldn't even do that in its *own* country: policy was, and always had been, that the CDC had to get an official invitation from a state or local public health agency before it could send out any of its people into the affected area. That was doubly true when you were heading off across the ocean.

There was the endless diplomatic trivia to worry about—the little matter of visas, for example. A Zairian visa was a rare commodity: you didn't just show up at the embassy and get one. Waiting periods of a week, Peters learned, were not uncommon. There were rumors of visa fees in the neighborhood of $150 or more, plus further "fees" (read "bribes"), if and when you made it as far as Kinshasa. Someone would have to coordinate with the State Department, with the World Health Organization in Geneva, with the Belgian and American embassies in Kinshasa, with Tamfum Muyembe and Julia Weeks.

And then there was the matter of collecting together the necessary supplies, shipping them off to Africa, and getting them there safely. The rescue team would need surgical gloves, gowns, rubber boots, duct tape, face masks, bleach, and body bags, among other items. Some years previously, in 1988, the CDC had printed, in a special issue of *Morbidity and Mortality Weekly Report*, a procedures manual for dealing with hemorrhagic fever outbreaks. It was called "Management of Patients with Suspected Viral Hemorrhagic Fever" and had been put together by Peters's predecessor at Special Pathogens, Joe McCormick. Peters knew the guidelines well enough, but he went through them again anyway.

"Double gloves, caps and gowns, waterproof aprons, shoe covers, and protective eyewear are required," the report said. Everything that came into contact with the patient—linens, pajamas, whatever—had to be "double-bagged in airtight bags. The bags should be sponged with disinfectant solution and later incinerated." The patients themselves "should be isolated in a single room with an adjoining anteroom serving as its only entrance. Hand-washing facilities should be available in the anteroom, as well as containers of decontaminating solutions."

Then there was the section entitled "Handling of a Corpse."

"All unnecessary handling of the body, including embalming, should be avoided. The corpse should be placed in an airtight bag and cremated or buried immediately."

That's the kind of stuff they were dealing with here.

Zaventem, the Brussels airport, was about ten miles east of the city. The terminal was very much in the European modernistic tradition, which was to say that it was spotless, hard-edged, and brightly lit. It was a world apart from the military cinder-block architecture of N'Djili, the international airport of greater Kinshasa.

Sabena flight 556 from Kinshasa touched down at Zaventem about 6 A.M. Brussels time, Saturday, May 6, taxied to the terminal, and pulled up to a gate at the international arrivals pier.

Carrying the little "frigo" box, the refrigerated picnic cooler containing the blood samples, Claudia left the plane along with everyone else. She walked through the Jetway, up a flight of stairs, and then emerged out onto the main concourse of the international arrivals pier. The concourse was at least a quarter of a mile long and straight as an arrow, glossy pink granite flooring the whole way, a row of perfectly white columns on either side that seemed to merge at infinity, the whole long passageway brilliantly lit by long, thin fluorescent tubes that ran the entire length of the ceiling. A moving walkway ran down the middle of the corridor, and the arriving passengers headed right for it despite their having been immobilized in airline seats for the last eight hours or so. Claudia stepped onto it, too, and rode along in silence.

Finally she came to passport control, where there were long lines. But Claudia, who was an experienced traveler, had no problem there. Customs, however, was another thing. Customs was where people got stopped for bringing in more modest contraband, items that were a lot less damaging than a twelve-pack of slightly lethal human pathogens. But she was passed through customs like a dream and suddenly she was free.

She came out into the wide main terminal where a crush of people stood behind a long silver railing—the friends and relatives of the arriving passengers. Her instructions were to look for a Dr. Johan van Mullem, whom she didn't know in the least. Dr. Lahaye in Kinshasa had called van Mullem the day before, alerting him to the incoming samples; supposedly, van

Mullem would be there in the crowd holding up a board with her name on it.

Claudia looked along the line of faces. She saw her name on a placard and walked over to the man holding it up. "Here are your viruses, Doctor," she said, handing him the box. "And I haven't had the slightest problem with customs." At which point Claudia retired forever from the biological-courier profession.

Johan van Mullem got into his car with the frigo box and drove out of Zaventem. He worked at the Brussels headquarters of the Belgian Development Cooperation, whose offices were at 6 rue Bréderode in the center of town, in a posh section right behind the Palais Royale. This being Saturday, however, the offices were closed, and so he took the samples instead to his home.

Van Mullem lived in a high-rise apartment building near Louvain, a few miles from the airport. He took the elevator up to the seventh floor, bringing the sample box with him, unlocked the door to his apartment, and put the box down in his living room. At that point, although no one in the outside world knew it, the fourteen Kikwit blood samples were cooling their heels on the seventh floor of a large residential dwelling in the Brussels suburbs.

At about 8 A.M., van Mullem placed a call from his home to Simon Van Nieuwenhove. Van Nieuwenhove was a colleague of van Mullem's at the Belgian Development Cooperation. He was in charge of the medical projects funded by their Central Africa Service, and he, too, was an old hand with Ebola, having been at both the Yambuku outbreak in 1976 and the Sudan epidemic in 1979. He'd been keeping tabs on the Kikwit situation since first hearing about it a couple of days earlier from Soeur Ignace, a Catholic nun who had run the Kikwit hospital's pharmacy for many years, but who'd since retired to Héverlé, also in the Brussels suburbs. She, in turn, had heard about the crisis by a late-night fax direct from Kikwit.

Van Nieuwenhove now left for van Mullem's place to pick up the sample box. He'd take it to Guido van der Groen . . . except for one minor detail. "It was Saturday morning," Van Nieuwenhove recalled, "and the Institute of Tropical Medicine was closed. It took quite a while to trace the private phone number of Professor van der Groen, but finally I got it and drove the samples to Antwerp."

Antwerp was about fifty miles away, and it took him about an hour.

"When the samples arrived on the sixth of May here in Antwerp," said Guido van der Groen, "I was extremely frustrated because in my mind I remembered the old history of about twenty years ago."

About twenty years ago, during the Yambuku outbreak, van der Groen's lab had gotten the very first specimens of Ebola ever to come out of Africa. He'd tested those samples himself and had seen the virus with his own eyes in the electron microscope. That, however, was the good old days.

"This time I could not do anything with them," he said. "I no longer had the proper biosafety lab, I no longer had the diagnostic tools to make a rapid diagnosis, and so I had to send them on to the CDC.

"So I did the following. I brought the samples to my lab. I opened the box, the plastic box in which the samples were, in order to see if everything was okay, in terms of not leaking. And then I froze everything."

He froze everything because it was by then too late in the day to round up some fresh dry ice, repackage the samples, and send them back out again. On the other hand, the next day, Sunday, was even worse: on Sundays everything in Belgium was shut tight as a drum. No dry ice, no Federal Express, no nothing. So the shipment would have to wait till Monday, May 8.

Except that Monday, May 8, was the very worst day of all.

It was a national holiday, V-E Day, celebrating the fiftieth anniversary of victory in Europe.

"We were commemorating the fact that Belgium during the Second World War was liberated by our American friends and our English friends—the victory over the Germans.

"To me it was not a victory," he added. "To me it was a hell of a day. The telephones were not working at the Institute, I could not make any phone calls, I could not send any fax. I could not even contact Federal Express. I was working in African conditions, and to me it was a hell of a day."

But he located some dry ice, repacked the box, got in his car, "and I began running the Ebola samples through Antwerp, trying to find the office of Federal Express." He'd never been there before and didn't know where it was in the city. Finding it at long last, he faced his greatest hurdle, which was filling out all the forms and getting the desk clerk to accept the parcel for shipment. This he did, he said, "by looking in a convincing way into the charming eyes of the young lady."

And then, from his wife's office, he sent a fax to C. J. Peters. The package, he said,

was sent BILL RECIPIENT.
The parcel will arrive +/– 10.30 local time in Atlanta on 9 May 1995
(according Federal Express).
Please confirm good receipt and keep me informed?
Do you have antigen-capturing ELISA for EBOLA?
Best regards
GUIDO

2   The Agency

At the time of the Kikwit outbreak, the Centers for Disease Control had attained the ripe old age of almost fifty years. Long before reaching that milestone, however, the CDC had become the symbolic world headquarters of the Men-against-Microbes movement. All over the world, whether they were in Casper, Wyoming, or Lassa, Nigeria, when public health officials confronted an otherwise intractable microorganism, they ended up calling the CDC because if they couldn't help you out, then no one could. So you called the CDC for advice and counsel—and also for permission to send in a wee sample of your problem microbe, whatever it was. Soon you'd get an answer back identifying the bug, telling you how to deal with it, and how to prevent that particular viral, bacterial, or rickettsial pest from ever rearing its ugly face again.

If you needed on-the-spot help, they'd send it to you without delay: actual live CDC disease militiamen were known to show up in a matter of hours, or days at the most. If you needed some biological reagents or testing materials or some viruses to experiment with, well, they'd send you that, too.

That's what the CDC was for, that was what it was all about. It was the Lab of Last Resort, it was the Home of All the World's Viruses and Bacteria, it was the hub of the planet's disease-fighting forces.

But it was far more than that, and as its fiftieth birthday approached, it had assumed the status of a vast and bloated government bureaucracy. It employed a grand total of 7,000 people in 170 different occupations from floor swabber to program head, a massive army of health workers spread out across the country from Anchorage, Alaska, to San Juan, Puerto Rico.

There were eight separate CDC facilities in the Atlanta area alone, with a colony of 4,600 federal health personnel spread out in office parks, industrial centers, and labs in Buckhead, Chamblee, Corporate Square, Executive Park, Koger Center, Lawrenceville, and Tucker. But whenever you heard the name "the Centers for Disease Control in Atlanta" on the nightly news or read it in the paper, what that phrase normally referred to was main headquarters, a complex of a dozen or so interconnected buildings located at 1600 Clifton Road in a semiresidential neighborhood a couple of miles east of the city.

From street level, 1600 Clifton Road was rather unprepossessing, wholly too small and plain to house this grand and legendary health establishment. It was a single six-story building, six long strata of windows and red brick that might conceivably house the department of motor vehicles or a branch of the social security administration, it was that bland and boring.

But the building was perched on a hill, and the ground fell away in back of it in such a way that the bulk of the place was actually below eye level. There was in fact a whole small city down there behind it, a maze of laboratories and specimen freezers, animal rooms, and endless offices. Some of those offices, indeed, were located *in* the animal rooms—former animal rooms, converted to work space—which had once housed caged monkeys, rabbits, rats, and the like. Such rooms were totally windowless except for a little peek-in square of glass in

23

the door through which the animal handlers had snooped on their captives. To gain some slight sense of privacy, the new human occupants blocked out the window with brown paper, tinfoil, or whatever. They could do nothing much about the little rectangular vent spaces at the top of the door, though, which at least provided some needed ventilation. There was also a three-inch-wide lip of concrete that ran completely around the animal-room offices at floor level, at the juncture where the wall met the floor. Originally, this was to keep water from collecting up along the seams while the janitors were hosing down the rooms during cleaning. Nowadays it mainly served to keep the human worker from pushing his or her desk, file cabinets, or bookshelves flush against the wall.

Still, these were minor inconveniences that never very much bothered the occupants.

"I run a bureau of four hundred people from the animal house," said Brian Mahy, director of the viral and rickettsial diseases division, whose office was in Building 6, which still housed some nine thousand animals—mice, rats, and rabbits mostly—plus a smaller number of humans. "It isn't a problem."

Also not a problem, once you got used to it, were the initially mystifying aboveground "subbasements." Half of the CDC's offices, it seemed, were in basements, subbasements, or *sub*-subbasements, most of which were located high above ground level. Anyone who climbed out of a basement window of Building 15, for example, would be in free fall for two full stories before ever hitting the pavement. But that's what happened when you kept adding on buildings rearward from the back slope of a hillside while leaving all the floor numbers constant.

It's also what happened when you underwent a boom period and built, populated, and reshuffled office space willy-nilly, which was pretty much the story of the CDC. It was a place that had started small and grew explosively, in both form and function. Indeed, its mission had expanded from modest and well-defined beginnings to a set of goals that were so nebulous and grandiose as to be almost unattainable by human effort.

And then, just at that very apogee of an all-embracing health utopianism where nearly every physical, mental, or other human ill, not excluding "violence," would be addressed and rectified through its work, the CDC's ambitions shrunk back under the combined weight of AIDS, African hemorrhagic-fever epidemics, and outbreaks of more homegrown diseases such as hantavirus, *Legionella,* and tuberculosis.

Naturally, like their kith and kin at every other government facility from the Pentagon in Washington to the post office in Scratch Ankle, Alabama, CDC officials will tell you regularly that they need more money. This was their never-ending mantra despite the fact that by fiscal year 1994 the agency was spending itself through a budget that topped $2 billion per annum, an amount larger than the annual budget of South Dakota, larger in fact than the gross national product of such developing countries as Guyana, Suriname, and Mauritania. But the CDC had been a casualty of mission creep and domain expansion, and whereas it had once targeted itself single-mindedly at the goal of eradicating human diseases—or at least controlling them—its ambition ultimately blossomed into a full-blown and all-purpose health megalomania.

"The mission of CDC is to promote health and quality of life by preventing and controlling disease, injury, and disability," said an official CDC publication. "The agency pursues improved quality of life for all by promoting healthy behaviors and lifestyle choices and fostering healthful environments."

The CDC's origins went back to an era before such terms as "quality of life," "healthy behaviors," and "lifestyle choices" were allowable in polite company. In fact, its earliest ancestor was a 1942 government agency devoted to the specific and sole purpose of controlling malaria in the southern United States.

Malaria was a disease characterized by sudden fever, chills, and sweats, along with weakness, lethargy, headaches, violent bodily shaking, and in some cases death. The ailment went back to ancient times, and the major symptoms had been described by the Greek and Roman medical writers, who even then associated the illness with marshes and swamps. Malaria—the very word meant "bad air"—was also associated with military service, for soldiers often went off to war in exotic locales in Africa, India, and the Far East, all of which were major strongholds of the disease. Indeed it was a French military surgeon, Charles Laveran, who in 1880 while stationed in Algiers discovered the cause of the illness to be tiny, one-celled parasites of the genus *Plasmodium*. And it was another military surgeon, Ronald Ross, who in 1897, after having been stationed in Burma, discovered that the parasite was carried by the *Anopheles* mosquito, which injected the microbe into human hosts in the process of biting. From all this the conclusion seemed to follow inescapably that if you could control mosquitoes, you could control malaria, thereby saving your fighting forces from at least one superfluous agent of death.

It made good sense, then, that within six months of the attack on Pearl Harbor, the surgeon general of the United States, Thomas Parran, established a national organization whose purpose it was to control malaria in the Southern states, which were a main troop training ground for the U.S. Army. The organization would be located in Atlanta, Georgia, a state whose many square miles of swampland made it a prime breeding ground for mosquitoes. Supposedly, it would be known as the office of National Defense Malaria Control Activities.

That was the name Parran proposed in February 1942, and it lasted for all of a month or so. He soon shortened it to Malaria Control in Defense Areas, and then, in April, changed it again, to Malaria Control in War Areas, MCWA, which is what the agency officially became. The "war areas" wording was somewhat puzzling in view of the fact that the agency's only mandate was to control malaria in the southern United States, whereas in truth the region hadn't been a "war area" since Lee surrendered at Appomattox. But it wouldn't be the only time the CDC would have identity problems.

The MCWA set up shop on the sixth floor of the Volunteer Building on Peachtree Street and plotted the eradication of malaria throughout the South. Soon some four thousand MCWA mosquito fighters were spraying tremendous quantities of various insecticides—DDT, diesel oil, and a poisonous green substance known as Paris green—at the offending bugs all over the Southern states, everywhere from southern California to Puerto Rico and the Virgin Islands. The effort was so successful that toward the end of it public health officials began to think in terms of eradicating the disease entirely. If that happened, of course, the office of Malaria Control in War Areas would have sprayed itself out of existence. Faced with that dire prospect, the health authorities responded in time-honored bureaucratic fashion, by expanding the agency's original charter to embrace items not previously included, using as justification the undeniable fact that lots of other diseases were out there that hadn't yet been attended to. This was a seemingly failsafe tactic, one that several CDC directors would self-consciously, and quite successfully, avail themselves of again and again. After all, no matter how many diseases the agency had already taken under its wing, another one was always waiting for attention. Any new disease outbreak, furthermore, could be turned into proof that the CDC was not yet big enough, and into an opportunity for making additional funding requests.

"We took advantage of every crisis," said Justin Andrews, the third of CDC's numerous chiefs. "When Asian flu came along, we were at the door asking for more money. When the staphylococcus scare appeared, we asked for more money and got it."

First to appreciate the fertility of this approach was one Joseph W. Mountin, M.D., an official of the U.S. Public Health Service. At an MCWA staff meeting a week after V-E Day, he said, "I don't say it to be throwing a scare into you folks, but we must look forward to the time when the war ends."

He himself had been looking forward to it for a while—since 1942, to be exact—at which time he'd come up with the idea that this little malaria-control outfit could be turned into something far more encompassing. After all, returning servicemen would bring home with them lots more than malaria, together with that other prime hazard of the soldierly life, venereal disease. They'd also bring back everything from typhus to dengue and yellow fever, tropical delights that most civilian physicians were ill-equipped even to recognize, much less cure. Why not set up some training programs, some infrastructure? Beyond that, and further into the future, he imagined a far-flung government health bureaucracy whose purpose would be to attack infectious diseases of all types.

He'd start with humble beginnings, though, with an unpretentious follow-on to MCWA. The new entity would be called the Communicable Disease Center and would concentrate on helping the states deal with a variety of local health problems. Congress would have to fund this new project, but who in the House or Senate could resist, especially after Mountin and his men went into action handing out photographs of MCWA sprayer-equipped jeeps rolling through peaceful suburban streets and parks, protecting Southern belles and fine American males from the *Anopheles* mosquito. It would be like voting against God or nature.

And so on July 1, 1946, the office of Malaria Control in War Areas was formally and officially deactivated as having completed its business. Malaria, indeed, had at that point virtually disappeared from the United States. But on that same day, the new Communicable Disease Center, the CDC, arose in its place. With any luck, it could do with communicable diseases in general what its predecessor had done with malaria.

The weird part about the Kikwit outbreak was the way the pathogen, whatever it was, seemed to appear out of nowhere.

One day it wasn't there, the next day it was. But that was normal routine for infectious diseases. "These things are always there below the surface," said C. J. Peters. "They just pop up from time to time."

Still, the question was, why did they pop up when and where they did? While the emergence of a given disease might look, from the outside, to be a chance event, unknowable and beyond prediction, the fact is that there was an underlying logic to it all, a bunch of perfectly intelligible reasons and causes why whatever happened, happened. Indeed it was a fundamental presupposition of epidemiology—the science of epidemics—that the nature and occurrence of diseases were as understandable and amenable to analysis as anything else in the known universe. Natural laws covered everything from subatomic particles to the stars and the planets. Why shouldn't they also cover diseases?

"Natural laws govern the occurrence of a disease," said William Farr, a medical statistician, back in the mid-1800s. "These laws can be discovered by epidemiologic inquiry. And when discovered, the causes of epidemics admit to a great extent of remedy."

To conduct an "epidemiologic inquiry," you of course first had to know that an epidemic was in fact occurring—which was not so easy as it might appear at first glance. People were always getting sick and dying; that was part of life. How could you tell that an "epidemic" was in progress?

You had to have some sort of health-monitoring system, one that would establish a normal health baseline against which significant departures would stand out in bold relief. Such systems had been tried out in the past, but many of them had not been all that effective. Initially, back in the 1600s, doctors reported only deaths, and not sickness, to health authorities, providing them with only part of the picture. Later, when the reporting system was still voluntary, many physicians refused to cooperate on the ground that a person's medical condition was a private matter between doctor and patient. And even when accurate data was finally collected, often as not nothing was ever done with it: it was never analyzed, sorted through, or made sense of. It just sat there in a file drawer, dead as the victim.

A practical health surveillance system required data not only about deaths (mortality) but also about disease (morbidity). And it required that such data be forwarded to a central sorting point where it was sifted through regularly and systematically. Pockets of "excess morbidity" and "excess mortality," which were the polite medical expressions for such things, would then show up like blips on the health radar screen.

By 1925, the states were making weekly notifications to the U.S. Public Health Service on the incidence of selected diseases. Still, knowing that a given illness was occurring did not by itself do anything to stop the spread of it; for that, some sort of direct intervention was necessary. From a public health standpoint, the ideal solution was to keep a team of seasoned disease fighters on alert, a standing army of trained epidemic-fighters who were ready to go out on a moment's notice. They'd travel to where the sickness was breaking out, discover its cause, break the chain of transmission, and thereby put an end to it. In the early 1950s, the CDC's founding father, Joe Mountin, proposed a distant forerunner to such a thing: he called it an "epidemic intelligence service."

As he originally conceived of it, the main purpose of an epidemic intelligence service was not so much to stop a disease as it was to distinguish a natural outbreak from one that had been artificially induced, which was to say, purposely caused by an enemy agent. This was the Cold War period during which the idea of biological warfare was taken with great seriousness—and with ample justification. After all, there was no reason why germs couldn't be used as weapons, and in fact they were admirably suited to the task: they were small and invisible, many of them deadly, and they left no traces as to where they came from.

In 1950, Alexander Langmuir, one of the few working epidemiologists then at the CDC, described a range of biological-warfare assault strategies that would do credit to a whole later generation of medical-thriller writers. An area's food and water supplies, he said, could be seeded with lethal pathogens that were totally undetectable until after they'd already done their damage. Microbe-laden clouds could be sent wafting over downtown Cleveland where they'd rain down upon the noon-day lunch crowd huge quantities of anthrax, smallpox, polio virus, or God only knew what other noxious stuff. The worst of it was that the resulting infections would be perceived as natural and spontaneous events instead of as deliberate attacks caused by a foreign power. All the difficulties of knowing that a natural-disease epidemic was occurring were only compounded when the sickness in question was artificially induced but intentionally disguised to look like a natural one.

That was the problem to be addressed by Joe Mountin's "epidemic intelligence service," which would constitute a flock of trained medical spies, a cadre of secret agents who'd go out into the field and track the infection rearward to its ultimate source. They'd be the James Bonds of biological warfare, on the trail of health sabotage.

About a year after Mountin first came up with the notion, the CDC officially established the Epidemic Intelligence Service along the basic lines he'd proposed. The first formal class, which met in July 1951, consisted of twenty-two M.D.s plus one sanitary engineer, all of whom came to Atlanta for a six-week course in practical epidemiology. The basic principles were simple enough: a person with an infectious disease either contracted it from another victim or had acquired it from a separate nonhuman source; in either case, finding the source was a matter of tracing back through the lines of transmission and zeroing in on a point of origin. It was detective work in the truest sense, as you waded into a breaking epidemic and chased down the essentials of person, place, time, and opportunity, exactly as if you were hunting a criminal. Frequently, making a map was crucial to the task, and in fact one of the most famous investigations in the history of epidemiology had taken place in 1854 when a physician by the name of John Snow traced the course of the cholera epidemic back to its point of origin by plotting out the cases on a map of London.

Cholera was an incredibly fast-working and horrific disease in which victims could lose up to 10 percent of their body weight in a matter of hours—a two-hundred-pound man could drop ten or twenty pounds in an afternoon—through profuse watery diarrhea and vomiting. Cases were on record in which people woke up healthy and were dead by sundown. Death was caused by simple dehydration: the victim just ran out of bodily fluids. Back then, physicians attributed the condition to "miasmas"—mysterious emanations from the ground—foul vapors, evil humors, and suchlike.

John Snow took a map of London and marked where each of the victims had lived. The pattern that emerged showed that five hundred cases lived within a few blocks of a public water pump on Broad Street. Whatever the causative agent, it was clearly centered on the Broad Street pump. Snow asked the city fathers to disable the pump so it couldn't be used, which they did by removing the pump handle, and lo and behold the epidemic receded within a few days. Only later was it found out that the pump had been drawing water from a source near a leaky sewer pipe, allowing seepage of the cholera microbe into the area's main water supply.

The CDC's Epidemic Intelligence Service soon forgot about biological warfare agents, none of which were ever discovered, and concentrated instead on outbreaks of naturally occurring diseases. The name Epidemic Intelligence Service was retained, but EIS officers changed from being disease spies in the biological-warfare sense to simple and basic disease detectives. That work was challenging enough, since nature's pathogens were far more cunning, covert, and mysterious than the average human enemy agent. In fact, that was a fundamental part of the appeal of such work: the mystery.

The Epidemic Intelligence Service soon developed into the functional hub of the CDC. Its main activities—disease surveillance and epidemic investigation—formed the whole essence of the place.

The Service's first chief, Alexander Langmuir, was a Harvard-trained physician whose uncle, Irving Langmuir, had been awarded the Nobel Prize for chemistry. Under Langmuir in the 1950s, the EIS would respond to any request for assistance, and officers from the unit could be counted on to show up at the local health department the day after being called in. EIS officers investigated outbreaks of bat-borne rabies in Texas, tracked contaminated polio vaccine in Illinois and California, and monitored smallpox cases during the WHO eradication program of the late 1960s. After a while, EIS people were being sent overseas, and a member of the unit had to be prepared to go anywhere in the world on short notice.

Forty-five years after its founding, none of this had changed very much except that the Service was now headed up by a thirty-six-year-old M.D. and Ultimate Frisbee champion by the name of Joanna Buffington.

By actual measurement, Joanna Buffington was just five feet one-half inch tall—"But I'm really taller than that!"—with a physique that she kept in fighting trim by never letting a moment go by without exercising. She rode her bike to work, she jogged during lunch hour, she rode her bike home and then went out for soccer practice, a Frisbee session, or maybe some running. She'd played soccer through high school and college and had been captain of the team for two years at Wesleyan.

She'd also gone out for gymnastics, track, and tennis and at one point had considered a career in exercise physiology.

She'd grown up in Massachusetts, where at age six she was initiated into biology courtesy of her buddy, Wretch Goodwin, who made a practice of blowing up frogs. He'd stuff them with firecrackers, light the fuse, and then stand back. Joanna was horrified, as was her mother.

To show him what he was actually doing, Joanna's mother caught a new frog and pithed it, severing its spinal cord, and dissected it in front of Wretch, Joanna, and the neighborhood kids. There it was, splayed out flat on the picnic table.

"Look, this is a living, breathing thing," her mother explained to the kids. "See the heart: it's still beating."

After which object lesson, Wretch Goodwin stopped blowing up frogs. "He blew up his sister Patty's plastic toilet from her dollhouse," Joanna said. "It was this great little toilet with a top that opened and a little flusher, and he blew that up instead."

Anyway, one thing led to another and Joanna grew up to be a full-fledged medical doc, specializing in family practice.

She hated it. She hated the patients who wouldn't take care of themselves, the smokers who came in with their fourth bout of pneumonia but who wouldn't quit smoking, the plump and portly jumbo types who wouldn't cut down on their eating, wouldn't exercise . . .

"I started to *resent* these people. And then I'd think, 'Wait a minute, a doctor is not supposed to feel like that. I'm supposed to be compassionate and caring.' But I was getting *angry* at these people!"

She even hated going in to the clinic. Matters came to a head one morning when she realized that she hadn't been wearing her seat belt for a week. "I thought, 'Do I want to kill myself?' Well, no, I just wanted to be hurt bad enough not to have to go in to work."

Any public health doc would totally understand the attitude:

by and large, physicians gravitated toward public health because they regarded traditional one-on-one medicine as boring, pointless, or both. Joanna's boss, hearing the seat-belt story, guessed that she was the perfect candidate for public health work. Public health, he explained, was a whole other way of doing medicine: the focus was on "herd health," which meant concentrating on groups of people rather than on individuals; the objective was prevention, immunization, making whole *populations* healthy.

Joanna ended up enrolling in the CDC's Epidemic Intelligence Service training program, which was essentially two years' worth of practical, hands-on education in discovering the origins of a breaking epidemic. Docs in training got a few weeks of formal instruction in the summer, after which they learned by doing, investigating outbreaks on their own.

There was the time that a nursing home in the Atlanta area was experiencing a bit of "excess mortality"—in other words, more people in the nursing home were dying than was normal. The question was, why? The nursing home's medical staff plainly was out of its depth—they didn't know what the cause was, the deaths had continued, and so they put a call in to the CDC.

Joanna arrived at the nursing home that same afternoon. She went through the facility, interviewed the staff, and took blood samples from the surviving patients. The deaths, she learned, were occurring on the skilled-nursing floor, which meant that the patients were bedridden and practically immobile. This was puzzling because in that case the infectious agent, whatever it was, probably wasn't spreading around by direct contact. So how *was* it spreading around?

While the blood samples were being tested, Buffington sorted through the data she'd collected, the basic facts as to person, place, and time: who died, where they'd been when they got sick, and the date and time when they'd first shown symptoms. Then she constructed what was commonly viewed as the chief

35

working tool of the practical epidemiologist: the "epidemic curve" of the outbreak. Basically it was just a graph of the data, but in visual form it told you a lot, especially in larger outbreaks, where you could see the successive waves of the illness, you could see what the incubation period of the disease was, and you could make some initial hypotheses as to the probable pathogen and how it was being transmitted from case to case.

So she made a graph in which the horizontal axis represented time and the vertical axis represented the number of cases that had occurred on each date. This yielded a histogram in which the height of a column showed the number of people who exhibited symptoms at each successive stage in the outbreak.

From these results, together with her questioning, it looked as if a single person was propagating the infection by going from bed to bed. Further delicate inquiries turned up the fact that one of the nurses on the "skilled-nursing floor" was known to be careless about washing her hands between patients. She'd go from one bed to the next without cleaning up in between, an extremely bad practice. The causative agent, the blood tests now showed, was parainfluenza, which for the nursing home's elderly and weakened population was a highly dangerous virus. End of mystery.

"Just getting more conscientious about standard infectious control methods was what put an end to it," Buffington recalled. "Washing hands between patients, that was the key to it all, and that's the most basic sort of prevention."

Time and again as she investigated new outbreaks, Joanna was amazed by the health value of simple cleanliness, and by the degree to which people flouted common sense on the matter. There was the hepatitis outbreak in Casper, Wyoming, for example. Hepatitis A was going around among some kids, and nobody could figure out where it came from. But it was not a pretty thing to see in a patient.

"You can get a little bit of a fever," Joanna said. "Stomach pains, headache, and jaundice. That's when people start noticing, *Gee, this kid looks yellow.* It's a liver infection and you get jaundiced and feel nauseous, have some diarrhea, your stools get light-colored, sort of clay-colored, and your urine gets really dark and you turn yellow."

So anyway she went out to Casper, interviewed the kids and the parents, including the first family to be affected. They, it turned out, had been on vacation near the Pine Ridge Indian Reservation about a month before the start of the outbreak, a time span that matched up perfectly with the incubation period of the disease.

Well, that's where it had come from, she thought: the Indian reservation. Hepatitis A was known to be fairly common among Native Americans; so prevalent was it on the Pine Ridge Reservation, in fact, that a new hepatitis A vaccine was undergoing trials out there at that very moment.

Further questioning, however, revealed that the vacationing family had never *gone* to the reservation. They'd just stayed at the resort nearby.

But *then* she learned that there was a hot tub at the resort. And she learned that some of the guests there, in a tremendous display of health consciousness and analytical intelligence, had been dunking their wee infants in the tub while their diapers were still on.

Dirty diapers in the hot tub! If there was a better way to spread hepatitis around, Joanna Buffington couldn't think of it. Disgusting as that was, Joanna had at least enjoyed solving the mystery.

Still, that puzzle was nothing compared to the *E. coli* case in Maine. A two-year-old had died in a hospital up there of hemolytic uremic syndrome, a rare kidney disorder one of whose symptoms was bloody diarrhea. The illness had been attributed to *E. coli* 0157:H7 bacteria, an organism that was particularly dangerous for small children, whose immune systems weren't yet fully developed. Currently in the hospital was a sibling of the child, exhibiting the same symptoms. Where had they gotten the bacteria from?

Buffington and another EIS officer, Paul Cieslak, went up to Maine and talked with the family. They traced the infection back to the kids' baby-sitter, who had herself experienced some of the symptoms and then recovered.

The baby-sitter, they suspected, had gotten infected on a farm she'd been staying at in New Hampshire. There were cows on the farm, some of them had been slaughtered and made into hamburgers, and undercooked beef was known as the classic vehicle for *E. coli* infections. The baby-sitter *had* to have picked up the bacteria from the hamburgers.

Except that the baby-sitter was a vegetarian.

Buffington and Cieslak now came up with a *second* theory, which was that the infection came from unpasteurized raw milk. Raw milk, they knew, was another classic source of *E. coli* infections.

So they went up to the farm and swabbed the cows and tested the milk . . . which bore absolutely no trace of *E. coli* bacteria.

Besides which, the baby-sitter didn't *drink* milk. "She didn't use *any* dairy products," Joanna said. "She was a strict and total vegetarian."

Then maybe it was the well water. Even a vegetarian had to drink water.

So on a cool fall day in October, Joanna Buffington and Paul Cieslak went back up to the farm and took more samples. They took water samples. They took blood samples from the cows. And then, just to be sure, they went around with Q-Tips swabs, picking up random tidbits here and there, anything that looked even remotely suspicious. "We swabbed the chicken coop, we swabbed the chickens, we swabbed just anything we could find, including the vegetables in the garden."

The irony was, it was the vegetables: they'd been fertilized with cow manure that contained *E. coli* bacteria. The baby-sitter had served and eaten the vegetables without adequately washing them first. Why people couldn't simply *wash things*—that was something Joanna never knew.

Back up in Maine, though, she'd felt very much like the complete disease detective.

"This is great," she'd thought to herself as she traipsed around the farm looking for samples. "Clear blue October sky . . . beautiful day . . . I've got these little sample bags, and we're trying to find something."

Never in her wildest dreams, back then, did Joanna Buffington imagine that she'd one day become involved in the most publicized disease outbreak of the late twentieth century. But by August of 1995, she, too, would be in Kikwit.

3   "This Is the Big One"

The Kikwit samples arrived in Atlanta on Tuesday, May 9, the day after Guido had sent them from Antwerp. The package was delivered to the receiving dock in the subbasement of Building 1 (which was at ground level), at 8:41 that morning. Tom Ksiazek, laboratory chief of the Special Pathogens Branch, came down to the dock and got them.

They were in a plain cardboard box about two feet on a side, which according to the airbill weighed 10.7 pounds. The airbill was marked: "DANGEROUS GOODS. Infectious substances, infectious to humans." At the Centers for Disease Control, this was the sheerest routine; they got scads of such parcels every single day of the week.

Ksiazek picked up the box and walked across the parking lot to Building 15, stuck his magnetic card into the card key reader, and took the elevator up two flights to his office in the "basement."

Building 15, the so-called Viral and Rickettsial Diseases Laboratory, was its own little realm at the CDC. It was the newest building on the premises, opened in 1988, and was all stainless steel and ceramic tile. It was like a space station in there, cool and quiet—except for the constant background noise, the sound of the fans maintaining negative air pressure, the viral hiss.

Ksiazek and Pierre Rollin, chief of the pathogenesis section, dressed themselves in gown and gloves, took the package into the P3 lab—biosafety level 3, less secure and stringent than level 4, which was maximum containment—and opened the outer cardboard box. Inside was a Styrofoam shipper, and inside of that, packed in dry ice, was a metal canister. Ksiazek opened the metal canister, within which, in Ziploc plastic bags, were the frozen vials of whole blood.

Ksiazek inspected them for damage, but all the tubes were still intact. Without opening them, he read off the data from each one—patient's name and the date the blood was drawn—and entered it all into the computer system. Then Pierre Rollin climbed into his space suit, picked up the samples, and went through the air lock into the biosafety-level-4 (BSL 4) lab, the maximum containment suite. The BSL 4 lab was hermetically sealed and so far away from the rest of the world that it was as if he was no longer in Atlanta.

Rollin defrosted the samples and aliquoted them out, dividing them up into smaller portions. He put some of the aliquots aside, then irradiated the rest with gamma rays, the purpose of which was to kill the virus so that the sample would no longer be infectious. Then he could work with them outside the space-suited confines of the maximum containment lab (MCL).

"There is no reason to run the tests in the MCL after you've irradiated the samples," Rollin explained. "You work much better when you're on the outside."

Pierre Rollin left the MCL with a rack of vials, brought them into room B105, a biosafety-level-3 lab full of computers, incubators, centrifuges, the standard complement of lab equipment, and handed them over to Mary Lane Martin.

41

Mary Lane Martin was a precise and placid research microbiologist who'd been at the CDC for twenty-nine years; in fact, she was within a year of retirement. She'd been born in Covington, Georgia, about thirty-five miles east of Atlanta, and she spoke with a strong Southern accent. In 1967, just a year after she'd come to the CDC, she'd worked with the original Marburg specimens, the ones that had come from the infected monkeys and humans in Marburg, Germany, the ones that had started the whole viral-hemorrhagic-fever era.

Mary Lane Martin got the samples at about two-thirty in the afternoon and started preparing them for an ELISA test. ELISA stood for "enzyme-linked immunosorbent assay," of which the basic principle was straightforward. You added a sample of the unknown virus to an enzyme that reacted chemically only to one specific virus and not to any others. A given enzyme, for example, would react only if you added Marburg virus to it but not if you added Lassa or Ebola or Crimean-Congo or anything else. In the presence of the right virus, the enzyme would turn a particular color, otherwise it would remain unchanged. This extreme selectivity of the reaction, the fact that a reagent would turn a given color with one and only one virus, allowed you to positively identify an unknown agent.

You could do this kind of test in the kitchen, provided you had the right enzymes, which was the crux of the whole procedure. This was why, in his fax of the day before, Guido van der Groen had asked C. J. Peters: "Do you have antigen-capturing ELISA for EBOLA?" Asking that question of the CDC, however, was like asking the Federal Reserve System whether it had banknotes. If there was anything that the CDC had an ample supply of, it was diagnostic reagents for the world's major and minor viruses.

And so, along about three o'clock on the afternoon of May 9, Mary Lane Martin took a prepared plastic plate and started dispensing measured amounts of the Kikwit samples into the ninety-six dimpled wells of the plate. The actual execution was somewhat intricate and involved a good bit of mechanical skill and practical know-how, and the various different reagents had to be deposited in the right order, washed off again, then mixed with something else, incubated, et cetera. Among the required ingredients were skim milk and horseradish peroxidase.

It wasn't until about three hours later, at about 6 or 6:30 P.M., that it was time to add in the last reagent, the telltale chemical, the one that would turn the sample wells green if they contained Ebola virus, but not otherwise.

Tom Ksiazek and Pierre Rollin were in there now, too, watching as she positioned the pipette tip over the sample wells and then pushed the plunger, releasing the chemical.

"I could see immediately when I added the last reagent that it was going to be positive," she said. "It started the color change almost immediately. I knew right away that they were going to be positive."

One by one the sample wells were turning green.

"God, look at that!" said Tom Ksiazek. "Look how many of them are positive!"

Pierre Rollin went out the door and came back a minute later with his camera. He took a couple of shots of Mary Lane Martin as she held in her lap the little four-by-six-inch plastic plate, the wells turning various shades of green.

The color of Ebola.

Three years after its resurrection as the Communicable Disease Center, the old MCWA was doing a lot more than controlling malaria. It was teaching personnel from state and local health departments how to deal with tropical diseases in returning servicemen. It was providing disaster relief in Texas after a series of chemical explosions in the state. It was making "health films" and other visual aids for use in its training courses in the United States and overseas. It was converting the abandoned Veterans Hospital at Chamblee, Georgia, into a laboratory.

The CDC now had its own library and credit union—even an insect museum. It had outgrown its Peachtree Street lodgings and spilled over into a total of thirty-five buildings in Atlanta, Montgomery, and Savannah. But an organization on an upward growth curve of this magnitude naturally wanted even more space, not to mention a proper headquarters, neither of which were in the offing as far as Congress was concerned. Nevertheless, support was immediately forthcoming from another source, albeit one that was wholly outside the confines of government. But who in their right mind, who in their most lurid fantasies, could have imagined that this growing government health machine, this paragon of public well-being and wholesomeness, would be helped out of its jam . . . by the president of the Coca-Cola Company?

Coca-Cola was a Georgia institution. Incorporated in 1888 with headquarters in Atlanta, it would be ruled over by one Robert W. Woodruff for more than sixty years. Woodruff was a brusque, independent-minded sort who had gone to Emory College, the predecessor of Emory University, for a brief spell on a unique proxy arrangement whereby he paid other students to do his homework for him. "If you can get somebody to do something better than you can do it yourself, it's always a good idea," he explained.

Early on in his Coca-Cola career, Woodruff had purchased the Ichauway Plantation, a private hunting grounds in Baker County, Georgia, abut two hundred miles south of Atlanta. Ichauway was a fabulous place, thirty thousand acres of pine forest, cultivated fields, and cattle pasture. Grazing upon its peaceful meadows was a palomino by the name of Silver, a horse that had been trained to guzzle bottles of Coke on command. Supposedly, it would never touch a Pepsi.

Woodruff often slept poorly and hated to be alone, so he would ask his guests to go out on horseback any hour of the day or night to hunt fox, turkey, dove, and quail, which were the plantation's major game species. Also residing at Ichauway, however, were staggering amounts of the *Anopheles* mosquito, carrier of the malaria parasite. At one point malaria was so common in Baker County that, according to estimates, some 60 percent of the population suffered from the disease. The first time he saw a case of the violent tremors it caused among his hired help, Woodruff was genuinely taken aback.

"What in the world is the matter with that fellow?" he asked.

"Malaria," he was told.

Shortly thereafter, Woodruff ordered a barrel of quinine pills—quinine was then the treatment of choice—for his hundred or so farm workers. He also put ads in the local paper offering quinine to any county resident who wanted it. Later, he donated money to Emory University so that it could set up a malaria research station at Ichauway, and he made another donation so that the college could purchase a fifteen-acre tract of land adjoining its main campus on Clifton Road and convey it off to the CDC. The CDC, Woodruff thought, had worked untold miracles with malaria control.

In 1947, the CDC bought Robert Woodruff's fifteen-acre gift tract for a token payment of $10. When, several years later, no actual buildings had yet appeared on the site, Woodruff jumped in again. Dwight D. Eisenhower, who was then president, had often hunted at Ichauway, and he and Woodruff were on a first-name basis. One day in the mid-1950s, Woodruff telephoned the president, who was on one of his frequent golfing holidays, in this case at Denver's Cherry Hill Country Club.

"Ike, do you have a pencil and paper?" Woodruff asked. "Why isn't the government putting up that CDC building in Atlanta?"

"Well, send me a note," said the president.

"I'm not gonna send you a note. I asked if you had a pencil and paper."

45

Shortly thereafter, according to the story, the whole long design and planning process was finally under way for real, all of it at Woodruff's personal behest.

He may have been closemouthed and secretive, and he may have smoked foul cigars, but Robert W. Woodruff, it seemed, was also a born philanthropist. "He had a strong aim to do good," said Bill Watson, a former CDC deputy director, who knew him.

By the time Mary Lane Martin got the Ebola results, the CDC's Kikwit team had been assembled and was ready to leave. It consisted of Ali Khan, Philippe Calain, and Pierre Rollin.

All three were M.D.s, but otherwise they didn't have much in common. Ali Khan had entered the Epidemic Intelligence Service program in 1991, graduated in 1993, then took up a position as medical epidemiologist in the CDC's Division of Viral and Rickettsial Diseases. He was currently the epidemiology chief of the Special Pathogens Branch, and at the advanced age of thirty-one had already been through several major disease outbreaks. The bulk of his work, though, had been in hantavirus, and he'd been at the CDC only a matter of weeks when virus broke out in the Four Corners area. Other isolated cases were cropping up here and there across the country, and Ali Khan flew all over the West investigating them.

He fast became an expert in shoe-leather epidemiology, going from house to house and interviewing people, blue backpack over his shoulder, little green notebook in hand. He investigated some ancient cases, solving puzzles that went back ten years or more.

"There was a case in Utah where a young woman's husband— he was a thirty-five-, thirty-six-year-old guy, with two kids—he was going along and doing his usual thing, and all of a sudden he got a fever, headache, muscle aches, didn't feel very well.

Within two days he was short of breath, and within three days he was dead, just like that. He died in the emergency room."

Nobody knew what the exact cause of death was, but the family physician had taken blood and tissue samples and stored them away for later identification. About ten years later, at the start of the hantavirus outbreaks in the Southwest, the doctor withdrew the samples from the deep freeze and sent them on to the CDC. It was Ali Khan who communicated the results to the family, telling them that the man had died of hantavirus.

"I was able to go back to them and say, 'This is why your husband died.' And the family—the father, the wife, the mother, the kids—they were actually relieved to hear this. They finally knew what happened. It sort of brought closure."

Ali Khan would be responsible for the epidemiology of the Kikwit outbreak. He had one major drawback for that enterprise, which was that he didn't speak French: "*Bonjour, bonsoir*, I think that's about the extent of my French. Oh, and *Bon dormi?*—'Did you sleep well?'" He'd need an interpreter the whole time. The other two team members, Philippe Calain and Pierre Rollin, would not have that problem.

Philippe Calain was born and educated in Belgium and had not only an M.D. but also a Ph.D. in virology. He was new to the CDC, having first set foot in Atlanta just two months prior to the Kikwit crisis. He was a small, bearded man, kindly and gentle, with a mien and manner that was so beatific that you pictured him as a Catholic monk in charge of the monastery's grape arbor. In Pavilion 3, the Ebola isolation ward, a different aspect of his personality would emerge—not that he knew, beforehand, that he'd be spending most of his time there. "I had no special instructions concerning my job in Kikwit," he said afterward. "I would have guessed I would have helped collecting blood samples, but we didn't yet know exactly what the situation was, who was already there, and so on."

On Sunday, May 7, Calain had been in the lab in Building

15, working on the genetics of hantaviruses, when Brian Mahy and C. J. Peters, who'd been holed up in the subbasement conference room, asked him to step in. They explained what they knew of the situation, that there was this big outbreak in Zaire, that it seemed to be connected with an operation performed in the Kikwit hospital on April 10, after which many of the operating-room personnel got sick and died. It could be Ebola, it could be Crimean-Congo hemorrhagic fever, it could be something else, nobody knew. Would Calain, as a native French speaker, virologist, and clinician, be willing to be shipped out there with the CDC team, departing sometime within the next couple of days?

Of course he would. He already had his full set of CDC background immunizations, he needed a shot for typhoid fever, and he needed to start in with a malaria prophylaxis, but other than for that he was ready to leave.

And then there was Pierre Rollin, a formidable presence by any standard. Rollin was big and tall, with a pair of wide-open, popping-out blue eyes that seemed to fix you in a cold gaze. He was Gallic to the core, with a fine sense of humor and wit, and from all outside appearances was a native Parisian, although he'd actually been born in Rabat, Morocco. He had a wife and four kids and had become an M.D. only because he couldn't get into veterinary school. "It's harder to be a vet than a physician in France," he said. "I missed an exam date, so I gave up and went to medical school."

At Montpellier University, the med school, he fell under the influence of a teacher who'd been at the Pasteur Institute, the microbiological research center located in the Montparnasse section of Paris, who made the place sound attractive. Rollin took some postdoctoral courses in virology at Pasteur and, in consequence, became wholly fascinated with diseases.

"My interest is in diseases as general systems," he said. "Not only the virus itself, but the disease in the patient, the pattern of transmission, the reservoir, the ecological cycle—what you might call, in the old-fashioned sense, the natural history of viruses."

He wound up as a research scientist at the Pasteur Institute, where he worked under Pierre Sureau. Sureau had gone to the site of the original 1976 Ebola outbreak in Yambuku, arriving at the hospital even before the CDC showed up. Later, Sureau and Rollin created a hemorrhagic-fever lab at Pasteur, which is where Rollin learned about working in hot labs.

At the CDC, Rollin lived on coffee, which he drank from an insulated mug that seemed to hold slightly less than a quart, and on the muddy jazz music that emanated from the CD player on his desk.

Pierre Rollin would be the leader of the CDC Kikwit rescue mission. Exactly what that would amount to, however, even he didn't know at the time, and in fact he was highly averse to advance planning under the circumstances. "If you go into an outbreak situation with a plan, you screw everything," he said. "My experience in African countries is, you go there and see what needs to be done, and you do it."

Not until 1960 did the Communicable Disease Center get a proper headquarters. By that time it needed one: the CDC had distributed itself out into a motley and disreputable collection of offices and government hand-me-down buildings—abandoned barracks, hospital wards, mess halls, and the like—none of which could exactly be called the pride of the public health service. In fact, many of them were dilapidated wood-frame structures that you lowered your life expectancy to enter, and some of the clerical personnel, not to mention the lab people, had contracted cases of the very diseases they were supposed to be controlling, making the whole thing something of a mockery. Offices were neither air-conditioned in the summer nor adequately heated in the winter. The animal facilities were not secure against breakouts, and monkeys routinely escaped from their cages, often wisely departing from the grounds without delay. It got so bad that at one point the CDC resorted to an officer-of-the-day system, one of whose functions was escaped-monkey retrieval.

From a health standpoint, the labs were off in their own special dimension of awfulness. "CDC's laboratories," said Elizabeth Etheridge, the place's official historian, "did not have germ-proof walls, individual-room air-conditioning, large-scale facilities for incubation, very low temperature refrigeration, or built-in hoods and inoculation chambers with exhausts and expelled-air incineration."

That's what the CDC did *not* have. What it did have were fifteen clear acres on Clifton Road in Atlanta, and grand plans for putting up buildings. Still, all those plans would have come to naught were it not for the support of the public health system's two congressional archangels, John Fogarty and Lister Hill.

Congressman John E. Fogarty was known as the Mr. Public Health of the U.S. House of Representatives. He was a Rhode Island Democrat who'd terminated his formal education upon graduating from high school, after which he'd become a bricklayer. So very many bricks did he lay that in 1936, at the age of twenty-three, he was elected president of the Rhode Island Bricklayers Union. In 1940, a mere four years later, he'd somehow parlayed that office into a congressional seat.

His later fixation on public health issues was a bit of a mystery even to him: "Nothing happened to me as a kid that made me decide medicine must be important," he once said. Nevertheless, as chairman of the House Subcommittee on Appropriations he lobbied for spending in the billions even while the officials of the Truman administration were plainly not interested in spending such lavish amounts on health. Fogarty had a counterpart in the Senate, though, with whom he teamed up to form a sort of public-health financing cabal, and between them they managed to get some rather substantial funding bills passed.

Fogarty's twin in the Senate was Lister Hill, Democrat from Alabama, the only state in the country that was even deeper South than Georgia. Hill's father, who was a surgeon, named his son Lister after Joseph Lister, the British surgeon who in the mid-1800s inaugurated the practice of antisepsis and who was later immortalized in the trade name Listerine. The measures Lister Hill proposed came to be known as Hill bills, and he is said to have sponsored a piece of legislation in which four thousand hospitals and health centers were to be funded in a single act of Congress.

Fogarty and Hill were chairmen of the respective House and Senate appropriations committees that oversaw health matters, and when they presided over public hearings on health spending, both men did everything possible to give money away, often at levels far exceeding those that the humble applicants themselves were prepared to ask for. The applicants appeared, hat in hand, to plead for a few spare dollars, when to their surprise baskets of untold cash were showered upon them.

Dr. William Henry Sebrell, director of the National Institutes of Health, once recalled what it was like appearing before Congressman Fogarty's subcommittee. "My testimony consisted essentially of being asked how much more did we need. Fogarty would ask the question: 'We understand that you are only allowed to ask for so much; if you didn't have that prohibition, how much would you ask for? How much can you effectively use?' "

Lister Hill was no different. When the witness was finished testifying, Hill would lean over the table and ask, in his best Southern drawl, "Are you shuah, Doctuh, that you're asking for enuff for these wunnnderful programs?"

With those two moneybags at the helm, it wasn't long before the necessary funding bills were passed—nearly $9 million had been appropriated—and the CDC's headquarters buildings were flying up at 1600 Clifton Road. There would be six of them altogether, spilling down the hill: offices, labs, auditorium and cafeteria, audiovisual facilities and soundstages, plus animal rooms galore. The place even had its own power plant.

This being the 1950s and Atlanta being the South, the new Communicable Disease Center also featured separate rest rooms for blacks and whites. The arrangement was much to the satisfaction of Lister Hill, who, despite being overflowingly liberal on public health matters, was a flat-out enemy of civil rights. In 1956, he along with one hundred other Southern congressional members signed the so-called Southern Manifesto, a document that criticized the Supreme Court's 1954 school desegregation decision as "a clear abuse of judicial power," which substituted "personal political and social ideals for the established law of the land." Later, Hill voted against the Civil Rights Acts of 1957 and 1960. Shortly after the dedication ceremonies in 1960, however, the tide had turned and the CDC's surplus rest rooms were converted into laboratories.

Other than for the rest room embarrassment and for the matter of aesthetics, never CDC's strong suit, the complex of buildings that finally arose at 1600 Clifton Road did credit to their two chief congressional supporters. All at once, the CDC had been turned into a reasonably modern medical institution. The whole place was air-conditioned, the research labs had the proper exhaust hoods and other accoutrements, and for the first time since it had been founded fourteen years previously, the CDC's physical plant seemed adequate to its task of controlling diseases.

Wednesday, May 10, C. J. Peters sent a fax to Terry McCulley at the Zaire desk of the U.S. Department of State, officially informing him that the viral agent in Kikwit had been identified as Ebola, suggesting that the Zaire officials be the ones to announce this, and asking that they do so immediately. "Any delay will be treated as a cover-up," he said in the fax. "Rumors about strange mutant viruses have already appeared and may spread panic."

Peters also had a question for Terry McCulley: "We have heard that there may be problems getting into Kinshasa. Are there any facts to this?"

Indeed there were. Zaire was not overly tourist-friendly, as was made clear by the "Consular Information Sheet" that the State Department's Bureau of Consular Affairs routinely sent out to prospective visitors to the country.

"Zaire is the largest sub-Saharan African country," it said. "It has substantial human and natural resources, but for the past several years the country has suffered a profound political and economic crisis which has resulted in the dramatic deterioration of the physical infrastructure of the country, insecurity and an increase in crime in urban areas (including occasional episodes of looting and murder in Kinshasa's streets), occasional official hostility to U.S. citizens and nationals of European countries, periodic shortages of basic needs such as gasoline, chronic shortages of medicine and supplies for basic medical care, hyperinflation, corruption, and in some urban areas, malnutrition of the local population to the point of starvation."

Visitors to Zaire, it further noted, could be expected to shell out certain "fees" for various imaginative but necessary "permits." "A government 'mining permit' may be required to travel to large areas of the country, regardless of the visitor's purpose in going there."

There was a last bit of news, about conditions in Kinshasa, the capital, which was just across the Congo River from Brazzaville: "There have been instances of shooting into Kinshasa from Brazzaville and of mortar shell fragments falling on Kinshasa from fighting in Brazzaville."

Shooting? Mortar shells? Bullets over Brazzaville? Even for

the most gung-ho CDC disease doc, live warheads were a bit unusual.

The next day, Thursday, May 11, the Zairian health officials made the formal announcement that the Kikwit outbreak was indeed Ebola. In fact it was a specific subtype known as Ebola-Zaire, one that was for all practical purposes identical to the strain that had broken out almost twenty years previously, in 1976, in the backwoods town of Yambuku in the northern part of the country.

Back then, nobody in the outside world had paid any attention: it was an isolated occurrence of an unknown disease off in the middle of nowhere, so who really cared? Things were a bit different this time.

Word went out first on the Internet, on various bulletin boards, discussion groups, mailing lists, and Usenet news groups such as bionet.virology, where the first rumors had appeared. On May 9:

Can anyone confirm that there has been a city recently isolated in Africa within the last few days due to a outbreak of Ebola? One person in our lab picked up something on the radio, but didn't get the full details. Would appreciate any further information.

That same day, a post came from within Zaire itself, from Paul Fountain, a doctor in Vanga:

!!!URGENCY IMPOSES!!!
I don't know if you are all yet aware of the virus outbreak here in our region. An epidemic surfaced, in Kikwit, Zaire, about 2 months ago. Until today there are 20 known deaths at the hospital with many more presumed in the residential quarters. Estimates run between 50 and 200 deaths so far.

People quoted various news stories that spoke of "fears that it may be the deadly Ebola virus, an incurable 'doomsday disease,'" and of "various villages that have been wiped out." A Zairian doctor was quoted as saying, "The situation could get totally out of control."

And so people on the Internet began asking certain obvious and pressing questions, such as:

Is Ebola virus the end of civilization?

Do killer viruses threaten the world?

Questions that were perfectly understandable. After all, Ebola was regarded as one of the deadliest viruses in history. When it had first emerged twenty years earlier, also in a hospital, the fatality rate had approached 90 percent. It was a fast-working virus; in some cases the victim was dead within a week after the first signs of the disease. So, when *Newsweek* ran a cover story entitled "Killer Virus," this could not be dismissed as an exaggeration: the name was literally correct and entirely true to the known facts.

This time, however, people paid attention. They were *bothered* by the fact that "the killer virus" had appeared, they were *scared* by it. And who could blame them? Hadn't Richard Preston written in *The Hot Zone* that killer viruses were nature's way of getting rid of human beings?

"In a sense, the earth is mounting an immune response against the human species," he'd said. "Perhaps the biosphere does not 'like' the idea of five billion humans. . . . The earth's immune system, so to speak, has recognized the presence of the human species and is starting to kick in. The earth is attempting to rid itself of an infection by the human parasite."

Worse, Preston's book had ended with the words, "It will be back," and suddenly there it was—the Ebola virus! It was back! The "coming plague" was *here!*

Nor, at least at first glance, did these apocalyptic conclusions seem wholly unjustified by the facts. After all, the general public had learned quite a few things about viruses by this point.

They'd learned, for one thing, that the common cold was caused by a virus, as was "the flu," or influenza. Those diseases were transmissible easily enough, by direct contact, or even through the air itself: somebody sneezed in a roomful of people—in a church, in a doctor's office, in an airliner, in the subway—and all at once everyone else in the immediate vicinity was infected.

This was not Stephen King or Michael Crichton. This was the way actual viruses operated in the real world: they floated through the air, got into your lungs, and a few days later you, too, had the disease.

And by now people had been told that in this respect the Ebola virus was just like the flu or the common cold: it, too, was transmissible by air. "A tiny amount of airborne Ebola could nuke a building full of people if it got into the air-conditioning system," Preston had written. "The stuff could be like plutonium. The stuff could be worse than plutonium because it could replicate." He'd even quoted C. J. Peters as saying, "We *know* it's infectious by air, but we don't know *how* infectious."

Late-breaking news reports, furthermore, had only added fuel to the fire. On May 10, correspondent Robert Bazell reported on the *NBC Evening News:* "Experts know the virus is transmitted by blood, but they worry that there may also be airborne transmission." And on that same day, the *San Francisco Chronicle* had quoted James Le Duc, of the World Health Organization, as saying, "If it is Ebola, this is the big one—this is what we're always thinking about when we talk about serious, dangerous disease threats."

This is the big one?

What could that possibly mean except that the Ebola virus was on its way to the United States, that it was getting ready to break out of Kikwit, emerge from Africa, its ancestral homeland, and arrive on your doorstep?

To many, the prospect was not outlandish. It was a modern

cliché of the jet age that any two points on the globe were now only twenty-four hours away. But what that meant was that the Ebola virus was now no more than twenty-four hours away from *you*. Your own home—your very own neighborhood—was only a day away from the Ebola virus!

The very worst of it, though, was when the world's public health officials started reassuring people, telling them that there was really no danger, that they didn't have to worry, that Ebola couldn't possibly materialize *here*. Hearing such stuff only confirmed your worst fears, because this is what public officials always did. The first thing they did whenever there was trouble on the horizon was to deny it; that was sure as the sunrise, it was absolutely dependable. They automatically denied things, covered them up, spin-doctored, whitewashed, backpedaled, and stonewalled. That was one of the major lessons of the twentieth century. Public officials could be counted on to do those things *especially* when all they were trying to do was to "prevent panic." Any American knew this instinctively.

So when those same Americans heard public officials minimizing the dangers presented by the Ebola outbreak ("the big one"), what exactly were they to think? The *Washington Post* quoted Ralph Henderson, assistant director-general of the World Health Organization, as saying, "The chance of someone getting on an airplane with this disease is just vanishingly small."

Vanishingly small!

That would have been comforting if only it were true. The fact was, however, that a person suffering from Ebola had *already* gotten on an airplane and flown to Switzerland, site of Henderson's very own institution, the World Health Organization. That had happened just six months previously, in December of 1994, when a Swiss primate researcher contracted the Ebola virus from a chimpanzee in the Ivory Coast. Unable to treat her properly in Abidjan, the doctors put her on a jet bound for Basel, Switzerland, where she was admitted to University Hospital.

So the Ebola virus, surprise, had already landed in Europe. It could easily come closer to home, for the virus had an incubation period that lasted anywhere between two days to three weeks, during which time the victim could be walking around in apparent health and never even be aware of the infection. The person could be sitting next to you on the plane, babbling away, quite chipper, the virus percolating deep in his body, replicating, duplicating, propagating itself like mad.

In fact, maybe it had already happened, because on May 18, there appeared on the Internet:

> ABC News reported tonight that a man was detained at the airport in Toronto who arrived on a flight from Zaire . . . he will be quarantined for three weeks to see if he shows signs of the virus. So much for the CDC's downplaying the chance of Ebola making it to our shores!

So if it could make it to Switzerland, if it could make it all the way to Canada, why couldn't Ebola make it to the United States? For all you knew, the goddamn virus had already landed in your own city.

For all you knew, maybe you were infected.

4 The Grand Arrival into Kikwit

A virus was one of the more remarkable entities in all nature. And in view of the damage it could do in relation to its size— a million viruses put together were about the size of a speck of dust—it exerted a magnetic pull upon the human intellect, an almost erotic fascination.

A virus was just a bit of genetic code, DNA or RNA wrapped up inside a protein coat, but that code held within it power enough to infect human cells, wreck bodily organs, kill plants, animals, and people, decimate populations, and demolish whole empires. That's what happened in 1520 when Hernando Cortés and a troop of six hundred Spanish soldiers invaded Mexico and met up with the Aztecs, who numbered in the millions. By rights, the Aztecs should have squashed Cortés and his men like bugs, but instead they themselves ended up dropping like flies. Cortés won his victory not by means of gunpowder, horses, or fabulous strategy, but rather by default, courtesy of a virus that he'd brought along with him, entirely unawares, to the New World. Aboard one of his ships was an African slave who had smallpox. The Europeans, having built up immunity to the disease through years of exposure, were safe from the virus. The Aztecs, by contrast, were a virgin population, had acquired no natural immunity to the disease, and died of smallpox as if the Spaniards had been broadcasting death rays.

All that was the work of a virus, which was essentially just an inert and dead chemical, a long-chain molecule of DNA or RNA, nucleic acids that had acquired the ability to enter a cell, take over its machinery, and compel the cell to make additional copies of the virus. The virus was able to accomplish this miracle because biological cells were all-purpose construction machines that produced whatever the incoming DNA blueprints told them to make. When left to their own devices, the cells went about their normal everyday business of reproducing themselves, making new proteins, and synthesizing the body's renewable constituents. Tiny molecular devices in the cells, the so-called ribosomes, followed the instructions contained in a given portion of the cell's own DNA and built whatever those instructions called for. If a certain DNA sequence coded for a specific enzyme, the ribosomes would read the sequence and synthesize the enzyme. If another stretch of DNA described a hormone, the ribosomes would read that stretch and build the hormone. And if still another DNA string described a virus, the ribosomes would read that string and synthesize the virus. Ribosomes were all-purpose construction machines, and as far as they were concerned, DNA sequences were DNA sequences, and one was as good as the next.

So when a virus infected a cell, the cell's ribosomes started building viruses instead of its own normal products, much as if an automated Toyota factory had been reprogrammed by an enemy agent and was now churning out Mazdas. That was why people died of viruses, because their cells were now producing alien substances instead of the person's own proper bodily parts.

One might wonder why it was that large and complicated organisms like human beings didn't have some sort of natural defense against viruses. But they did: they had the immune system.

The immune system was vast and complex, composed of macrophages, antibodies, and T cells, among other things. Macrophages were large, roving biological scavengers: they ate foreign matter and spit out the digested parts. They were completely indiscriminate in what they ate; they consumed anything in the body that didn't look like normal healthy tissue, including viruses, and turned them into so much innocuous trash. That was the first line of defense.

Then there were the antibodies. Antibodies were little Y-shaped molecular structures that floated around at random in the bloodstream and physically clamped on to foreign substances in such a manner as to render them harmless. They were like little hands or grippers that by virtue of certain chemical and structural qualities were able to recognize alien biological molecules, including viruses, grab on to them like the jaws of a bear trap, and immobilize them forevermore. That was the second line of defense.

All too often, though, viruses managed to evade both defenses, and some virus particles infected cells before either the macrophages or antibodies ever reached them. Then, inside the cell and safe from its adversaries, the virus could take over and do as it pleased.

The immune system, however, had a third line of defense, one that came into play in exactly this situation, where the virus was hiding out in a cell and taking over its internal machinery. The third line of defense was the killer T cell, so-called because its function was to kill those bodily cells that had already been invaded by viruses. In other words, it would destroy infected cells in order to destroy the viruses hiding inside them. This was somewhat like a country's bombing its own cities to kill the enemy soldiers who had stationed themselves within city limits: it was a strategy that would work, but only at an exceptionally high cost.

"If a virus multiplies and radiates quickly," said immunologist William E. Paul, "the immune system's attempts to contain it may do no more than leave a path of destruction in the wake of the virus, while never quite catching up to it."

Viruses, then, were highly noxious to living systems. Therefore, why not eradicate them? Why not get rid of them? Why not wipe them out, exterminate them, banish them from the planet?

During the 1960s, the Communicable Disease Center decided to get serious about eradicating at least one virus, smallpox, from the face of the earth. The idea was to remove it from nature. It was a notion that, had it first arisen thirty years later, in the 1990s, when people saw nature as rather aiming to eradicate humankind, would have been dismissed as the worst sort of lunatic-fringe delusion, as a quaint holdover from the halcyon days when people still believed in "impossible dreams." In the 1990s, anyone in his right mind would be expected to understand that eradicating lethal diseases, together with the virus that caused them, was a manifestation of that unpardonable sin called hubris.

In the 1960s, however, hubris was for the briefest instant actually chic. It was, after all, the time during which an otherwise sane and respected American president stated, in all sincerity, "I believe this nation should commit itself to achieving the goal, before this decade is out, of landing a man on the moon and returning him safely to the earth."

If that was not craziness, it was incontrovertibly hubris.

The sixties was also the decade by which diseases such as malaria and bubonic plague had been almost totally eradicated from within American borders, and with the coming of the Salk and Sabin polio vaccines, polio was clearly on its way out as well. As for smallpox, it was already extinct in the United States, and had been for some years, but it was still killing people in more than forty countries in South America, Africa, Asia, and in Europe. It was a disease that went back to antiquity, to ancient Egypt in fact, one that had caused disastrous epidemics for literally thousands of years and had been one of the biggest killers in human history, responsible for an average of 10 percent of all deaths each year. Smallpox was an extremely disfiguring condition that left permanent scars on those who survived it, sometimes also leaving them blind. Those who didn't survive died within one or two weeks, their bodies literally rotting away amid great stench and pain as the pustules covering the skin ran into each other and merged into large welts.

The disease had been contemplated as a biological-warfare agent as far back as 1763, when Jeffrey Amherst, commander in chief of the British forces in North America, suggested that one of his colonels, Henry Bouquet, create a smallpox epidemic among the Indians. "Could it not be contrived to send the smallpox among these disaffected tribes of Indians?" he asked. "We must on this occasion use every stratagem in our power to reduce them." The plan was to distribute smallpox-laden blankets to the tribes and then let nature take its course. Whether the plan was carried out is not known; smallpox, nevertheless, was highly lethal to American Indians, of whom it was estimated to have killed several million.

Even at mid–twentieth century there was no treatment for the ailment once you had it, and at the start of the 1960s smallpox was killing about a million people a year. On the other hand, smallpox was a virus that seemed tailor-made for a worldwide eradication program. Unlike many other viral diseases that were carried by animals or insects, the only known reservoir of the smallpox virus was the human race itself, meaning that if it was ever eradicated from the human population, there was no way it could come back from another source in nature. Once it was gone, it would be gone for good.

Second, smallpox was a scourge with a classic and extremely reliable preventive in the form of a vaccine. It was in fact the first disease ever prevented by vaccination, a practice that had roots far back in folklore long before its validity was scientifically tested by the British physician Edward Jenner in 1796.

By that year it was common knowledge that milkmaids rarely got smallpox. The reason, supposedly, was that they first contracted cowpox, a similar but milder disease, from the cows they milked, after which they were magically immune to both cowpox *and* smallpox, although no one understood why. In 1796, when a smallpox epidemic killed thirty-five hundred people in London and thirty thousand in the rest of Great Britain and Ireland, Jenner put the folklore to experimental trial. He found a milkmaid, Sarah Nelmes, who had cowpox, took some fluid from a blister on her hand, and deliberately infected a boy, James Phipps, with the serum.

Phipps came down with cowpox right on schedule. Two months later Jenner took the gamble of his life ("I could scarcely persuade myself that the patient was secure from Small Pox," he later wrote) and scratched some smallpox serum into the boy's skin. Not a winning experimental protocol in twentieth-century medical terms, perhaps, but anyway it worked. The boy was immune to the disease.

It was a case of artificially induced natural immunity. The procedure worked because the cowpox particles in the bloodstream provoked the body's immune system to start waging its many-pronged war, a battle that it won in this case because the cowpox virus was mild and slow-working enough to be controllable. Then, because cowpox virus molecules were structurally similar to smallpox particles, immunity to the one was also immunity to the other.

On the strength of this and his later successes with vaccination, Jenner claimed in 1801 that "it now becomes too manifest to admit of controversy, that the annihilation of smallpox, the most dreadful scourge of the human species, must be the final result of this practice." One hundred years later, smallpox had not been annihilated, although some countries had managed to eliminate it from within their borders. Sweden, the first to do so, had been free of the disease by 1895. Puerto Rico followed in 1899, Austria in the 1920s, England, the Philippines, and Russia in the 1930s, and Canada and the United States by the 1940s. But what could be done in each of these countries individually could also be done for the world as a whole, the final result being that through human effort and with malice aforethought, the smallpox virus, a large, brick-shaped molecule of DNA wrapped in protein, would be made absolutely extinct throughout the world.

By the mid-1960s, the Communicable Disease Center was part of the World Health Organization's grand plan to eradicate smallpox in ten years, starting in 1966. It was the quintessential public health project, a large-scale group effort aimed at inducing herd immunity, with the herd in question being the total population of planet earth. It was on a par with the moon shot, except there were no astronauts.

But the CDC didn't need astronauts; it had Prince Tungi.

Prince Tungi was the three-hundred-pound-plus maximum leader of the Pacific-island nation of Tonga. Tonga was a group of tiny islands some three thousand miles south of Hawaii and not near anyplace else, and its population of sixty-five thousand had never seen a case of smallpox, which meant that they were a virgin populace with no built-up immunity to the disease. The islanders, however, were now starting to export bananas and other produce to markets in Asia where smallpox was widespread, thus placing the nation at considerable risk of importing the disease, with fatal results.

So Prince Tungi came to Atlanta and was filmed by the CDC's movie crew while he was getting vaccinated with the newly developed "ped-o-jet." This was essentially a vaccine-loaded machine gun that had been invented by the U.S. Army to do vaccinations en masse. It had a stainless steel nozzle, weighed twelve pounds, was powered by a foot pedal, and could deliver a thousand doses of vaccine per hour in the form of a concentrated spray to the arm.

Soon, four CDC physicians with ped-o-jets and the all-important Prince Tungi film clip were in Tonga. Over ten weeks they went from island to island, showed the film clip again and again, and managed to immunize the whole population. All this was later immortalized in the CDC production "Miracle in Tonga," in which Prince Tungi himself played the starring role.

But Tonga, dispersed as it was, proved to be easy compared to wiping out smallpox in West Africa, which was the task allotted to the CDC by the World Health Organization. The CDC's Don Henderson, who had been the EIS chief, headed up the program; later he departed for WHO headquarters in Geneva to direct the worldwide eradication effort.

The CDC's goal for West Africa was "zero pox in five years," but it was not obvious from the start that such a timetable was realistic. Africa, the birthplace of humankind, was the bane of medicine, with the world's greatest elaboration of endemic and seemingly intractable diseases. Its countries had some of the world's highest rates of smallpox: in Sierra Leone, for example, the incidence was nine times greater than in India, which was itself a major preserve of the disease. West Africa was a vast area all by itself, with a huge population that would soak up more than 100 million doses of the vaccine, which would have to be administered in some of the remotest locations imaginable.

Plus there was the "playing God" problem. This was not the *ordinary* "playing God" problem, the one that scientists encountered whenever they wanted to usher in a major new change to the natural order of things: when they wanted to do recombinant DNA research, when they wanted to do gene

66

therapy, when they wanted to invent a new breed of mouse for research purposes, they were automatically accused of "playing God."

In the case of smallpox, matters were worse than that—far worse. There was, it turned out, *a god of smallpox*. In fact, there were many: in India it was the goddess Shitala; in Africa it was the god Shapona; in the New World—in Brazil and parts of Latin America—it was the god Omolou or Obaluaye, and when Desi Arnaz, the Cuban-born husband of Lucy in *I Love Lucy*, sang the fifties hit song "Baba Luaye," he was singing, whether he knew it or not, about Latin America's very own smallpox god.

In their respective cultures, the smallpox gods were thought to hold sway over the disease. They meted it out as punishment and they withheld it by way of reward, and so they could not be expected to look favorably upon doctors with ped-o-jets who were committed to wiping out the god's own pestilential kingdom. The believers in those gods, therefore, were highly dubious about the eradication exercise, and in fact when a CDC vaccination team landed in western Nigeria, they were met with drawn knives. "The word for smallpox in the local language was identical to the name of the local earth god," said Bernard Challenor. "The population was highly incensed, feeling they were being asked to make war on one of their own deities."

But by means of explanation, example, and persistence, all these problems and many more were surmounted by the CDC's vaccinators, who delivered a total of 25 million injections in a year's time, which put them a year and a half ahead of schedule. The feat was marked by music and celebration in Accra, Ghana, and Dave Sencer, chief of the CDC, flew in for the occasion.

The process only accelerated after that, as a result of two major technical advances. One was the bifurcated needle, which immediately supplanted the clumsy and bulky ped-o-jet.

Developed by Wyeth Laboratories, the bifurcated needle was a tiny tweezers that held between its two points precisely the right amount of vaccine. Anybody could be trained to use it: you jabbed a person's arm fifteen times in rapid succession, and that person was safe from the disease.

The second change was to the theory of how to create herd immunity. At first, the presupposition had been that to wipe smallpox off the face of the planet you'd have to vaccinate everybody in the world: that much seemed plain and obvious. But in the summer of 1967, Bill Foege, a CDC physician who was directing the immunization program in Nigeria, realized that universal vaccination was not in fact required to make a given population disease-free. The only ones you needed to vaccinate, he claimed, were those in danger of exposure from others. Those in no danger of exposure—pockets of people in a smallpox-free area, for example—didn't need to be immunized at all: they didn't need any "protection" because there was no threat to protect them against. So you'd do *selective* vaccination instead of *universal* vaccination, shooting the bullets toward where the culprits lay rather than firing them willy-nilly all over the place.

The key to the strategy's success was use of surveillance, the "health radar" system that CDC had put so much stock in over the years. You'd have to be on watch for isolated outbreaks of the disease in unvaccinated populations so that if and when the disease suddenly broke out among them, then you'd vaccinate all those likely to be in contact with the victims.

Within the CDC itself, this accelerated technique came to be known as eradication escalation, abbreviated as E-squared or E^2. Some people at WHO headquarters in Geneva didn't much care for the phrase *eradication escalation*, which reminded them of the "strategic bombing escalations" then taking place in Vietnam, and so in their fastidious and proper way they spoke instead of "surveillance/containment" and of "selective epidemiologic control."

Whatever it was called, Bill Foege's E^2 technique worked like a charm, and by May 1970, more than half the continent of Africa was smallpox free.

On Wednesday, May 10, four days after getting the call from Julia Weeks, Ali Khan, Philippe Calain, and Pierre Rollin—the CDC's Kikwit team—left for Africa.

Africa. In its own way it was the most otherworldly region on the face of the earth. It was wild, it was overgrown, it was foreign. And it was big: Africa was the largest separate continent, bigger than North America and almost twice the size of South America. You could drop the entire United States into it three times and still have room left over. Zaire, formerly the Congo, was itself immense—almost a million square miles, a territory larger than all of the United States east of the Mississippi.

Big as it was, the Congo was at one time the personal and private domain of a single individual: Leopold II, King of the Belgians.

King Leopold, by all accounts, was a man without quite enough to do. He had white hair, a long, stringy beard, and a hooked nose. Belgium, his "little kingdom," was only slightly larger than the state of Vermont, but it was moderately wealthy and heavily interested in international trade. Leopold was intent on acquiring a colony for his kingdom and had once offered to purchase the Philippines from Spain, but was rebuffed. (Spain sold the islands, all right, but to the United States, which in 1898 bought them for $20 million.) The Congo, however, was still available, having only recently been explored by Henry Morton Stanley, who successfully descended the Congo River in 1877. The only obstacle to Leopold's grand plan was that the Belgian parliament had no interest in acquiring colonies; if King Leopold wanted the Congo, he'd have to obtain it himself.

Which he did. In 1882, he formed the Association Internationale du Congo, a private trading corporation, and installed himself as head. He hired Stanley to return to the Congo and buy out the tribal chiefs, one by one, until the Association had clear title to much of the country. Stanley actually bought up the whole place, piecemeal, a parcel at a time, just as if he were the Donald Trump of Central Africa. He even wrote up a passably Trumpesque autobiographical account of his trading skills, boasting that by 1884 he was "in possession of treaties made with over four hundred and fifty African chiefs, whose right would be conceded by all to have been indisputable, since they held their lands by undisturbed occupation, by long ages of succession, by real divine right. Of their own free will, without coercion, but for substantial considerations, reserving only a few easy conditions, they had transferred their rights of sovereignty and of ownership to the Association."

King Leopold II was now in exclusive personal possession of an entity to which he gave the name the Congo Independent State. Since he'd acquired title to the land by paying out his own money, he conceived himself as actually *owning* the land, owning the whole country, as his very own personal property. He was, as he said, "the founder of the State; its organizer, its owner, its absolute sovereign. . . . My rights over the Congo are to be shared with none; they are the fruit of my own struggles and expenditure." He owned the Congo just like anyone else might own a place at the seashore.

He never once set foot in his private country. Rather, he sent out agents to harvest commodities—mainly rubber and ivory—for sale elsewhere. These agents had, soon enough, turned what could have been a peaceful system of paid labor and free trade into a realm of slavery and slaughter. The agents enforced production quotas by cutting off the ears, feet, or hands of the African workers who failed to meet them, and they stored the severed limbs in baskets. One basket was said to have contained 160 human hands; to preserve them against the heat and humidity, the body parts had been smoked over charcoal fires.

To stop these practices, Belgium took over the Congo in 1908, whereupon it became the Belgian Congo. King Leopold II died a year later. Belgium granted independence to the country in 1960, after which it was ruled over by Patrice Lumumba for a few months before he was murdered in 1961. Moise Tshombe became president for another short stretch, until the position was taken over in 1965 by Gen. Joseph-Désiré Mobutu. In 1971, Mobutu changed his name to Mobutu Sese Seko (meaning "the adventurous land"), changed the country's name to the Republic of Zaire, and ordered all those with Christian names to change them to African names.

The name changes did nothing to solve the country's economic and political problems, which were huge. Neither the roads nor the rule of law were maintained by the authorities, who seemed to have little control over the country they allegedly governed. Public servants often went unpaid for months at a time and made up the loss by theft, extortion, or other lucrative sports. It was no exaggeration to speak of the country as essentially in chaos.

This was the place to which Ali Khan, Philippe Calain, and Pierre Rollin were now headed. They'd left Atlanta Wednesday afternoon on a United flight to New York, then boarded a Delta flight that arrived in Geneva at nine o'clock the next morning. Traveling along with them were some fifteen trunks full of medical supplies from the CDC: disposable plastic gowns, aprons, face masks, rubber gloves, plus various items of technical gear including a satellite telephone and a computer.

They stopped in Geneva for about three hours, long enough to be driven to the local Zairian embassy to get visas, then back to the airport in time for a Swissair flight to Kinshasa. They also met up with Bernard Le Guenno.

Le Guenno was the Pasteur Institute's viral hemorrhagic fever specialist, a position that he'd acquired in 1983 after it had been vacated by Pierre Rollin. The two of them had worked at the very same lab, though never simultaneously. They were good friends, however, with congruent senses of dry wit, and in fact both of them had been within a couple of weeks of joining up in the Ivory Coast to investigate an Ebola outbreak that had occurred there the previous year, in November 1994.

The virus had broken out among a group of wild chimps in the Tai Forest, a wildlife preserve on the edge of West Africa. Primatologists had been in the area studying the chimps in their natural habitat for a decade. Every so often, but mainly at the end of the rainy season, the chimps would suffer an epidemic die-off of some sort. There had been one in November of 1992 during which eight chimps died over a two-week period. Two years later, in November of 1994, again at the end of the rainy season, there was another fatal outbreak. After performing an autopsy on one of the chimps, a thirty-four-year-old Swiss technician fell ill with a severe itchy rash, high fever, and acute diarrhea. Two days later she was transported to a hospital in Abidjan, the capital city of the Ivory Coast. Doctors there treated her with antimalarials, to which her illness did not respond.

That was not surprising because she was in fact suffering from Ebola, which she'd acquired from the dead chimp. She was flown out to Basel, Switzerland, where she recovered. Le Guenno and Rollin were about to embark on a two-week trip to the Ivory Coast to search for the reservoir, or natural host, of the Ebola virus that had killed the chimp when the news came of the outbreak in Kikwit.

At about 11:30 A.M. Thursday, Ali Khan, Philippe Calain, Pierre Rollin, and Bernard Le Guenno boarded Swissair flight 274 for Kinshasa. The plane made a stop in Libreville, Gabon, before arriving in Kinshasa at eight o'clock that same evening. It was a long flight, about eight hours of flying time.

N'Djili international airport in Kinshasa was not a place you wanted to disembark without the aid of competent professional services. The terminal was a concrete blockhouse packed to the gills with screaming people and gun-toting military men dressed in camouflage suits, all of them there for the sole purpose of fleecing the passenger: each of them demanded their fees before passing you on to the next in a long line. If you didn't know how to deal with this, you could easily drop $400 or $500 in the space of an hour. In Kinshasa, however, there were people who made a living at guiding you through the gauntlet in such a way that you paid the minimum. These fixers, who were said to be part of the so-called informal economy, themselves charged a fee for their services, but in the $100 range it was one of the greatest bargains in modern Zaire.

Lynette Simon, of the USAID office in Kinshasa, played the fixer's role when she met the CDC team at N'Djili and got them out of the airport in an hour or so. She took them to the only decent hotel in the city, the Inter-Continental. CDC people were public servants who traveled on a per diem basis, and the hotel was so expensive—about $200 a night—that they had to double up: Philippe and Ali in one room, Bernard and Pierre in the other.

They got rooms on an upper floor, went to the windows, and looked out. Down below the treetops they could see the swimming pools and the tennis courts, and the river Congo off in the distance.

The four of them gathered together in Bernard and Pierre's room and watched Zairian television—Tele-Zaire—on which there happened to be a story about the Kikwit outbreak. For a while it was just a voice-over in French with only the words "Communiqués and Messages" on the screen—it was like watching the radio—but then there was an anchorman and then some fuzzy shots of Kikwit, of the hospital, and then of

73

the Ebola virus itself. All of them recognized the picture: it was an electron-microscope photograph that had been taken at the CDC by Fred Murphy, almost twenty years earlier. It showed a single Ebola virus particle, one that had come from a dying nurse whose blood had been drawn in a Kinshasa hospital in October of 1976.

The next day they left for Kikwit. Although it was reputed to be a lost African backwater, the truth was that there were routine airline flights to the city. You even had your choice of services: there was the Mission Aviation Fellowship, which flew a single-engine Cessna back and forth to Kikwit; there was Air Kasai, which ran regular flights on a DC-3 for the one-way rate of $80; there was a competing airline called Air Malu; and there was a charter service named Air Excellence, which would fly you to Kikwit and back in a Beechcraft prop jet for the round-trip price of $2,500. All of them left from Kinshasa's smaller airport, N'Dolo.

N'Dolo was where the medics had the first of their many encounters with the press. The airport was crawling with journalists: there were Minicams, microphones, lights, tripods, camera bags, interviewers, soundmen, tape recorders, people in khaki vests studded with 35-mm film canisters. "Twenty journalists and only four scientists," said Bernard Le Guenno.

All of them climbed aboard the plane for Kikwit, the Air Kasai DC-3. The craft had been built in the 1940s, back before most of its passengers had been born. It was so old that there was a scantily clad female figure painted on the nose, just as if this were still World War II.

"Not very reassuring," said WHO's David Heymann, who'd taken the same plane two days previously. "That was the most fear I had in the whole outbreak. I don't like to fly in old airplanes."

But it staggered off the ground and headed east along the Congo. It was a wide river that flowed slowly, a sensation only increased by the altitude. Out the window you could look down and see scattered islands green with vegetation. You could see barges and steamers, large white multideck ferries carrying cars, trucks, and a thousand or so people, together with a number of assorted animals. You could see long, thin bark canoes—pirogues—being paddled along, slender wakes trailing off behind them.

The plane flew across flat, grassy savannas, stands of palm trees, muddy rivers that snaked back and forth. Here and there were some low hills, and spread out lengthwise along the hilltops were tiny villages, or at least clumps of houses and mud huts. Then it was all deep forest with glints of water shining up from the forest floor.

The flight took about an hour and a half. Then the plane banked and turned, and suddenly you were over Kikwit. You were finally seeing it with your own eyes, after three days of traveling and four separate airline flights.

You hadn't known exactly what to expect, beforehand. Kikwit had been described in the press as having a population somewhere between four hundred thousand, the size of Atlanta, and six hundred thousand, the size of Washington, D.C., and so you had this mental vision of a modern metropolis, of skyscrapers rising out of the mist, of a dense and teeming inner city.

But Kikwit was nothing like that. It was low to the ground and almost flat. There were palm trees, dirt streets, tiny homes spread out in grids. You could see farm plots, small ones, as if kept by single families. There were ravines, steep, sandy cliffs that went down to a river—the Kwilu, which bordered the city. As the plane got lower, you could see that the homes were actually brown wooden huts covered with rusted metal roofs.

The plane landed on a paved strip at the end of which there was a washed-out gray concrete building—was this the "terminal"?—with the word KIKWIT painted on the side in large letters. Standing next to it was a small crowd of people.

The four medics unbuckled their seat belts, walked down the

steeply sloping aisle of the plane, and looked out the back hatchway. And there at the bottom of the staircase, filling their entire field of view, wall to wall, were . . . Reporters! Journalists! Photographers! They were snapping away, taking pictures of the doctors like crazy, firing their Minicams, pointing them straight at them, at the Incoming Medical Saviors.

The journalists, who'd been in the plane with them, had burst out of the hatch like buckshot, like a blast of air, in a single rush, as if their very lives depended on it. They were facing the plane, taking a million pictures of Pierre Rollin, who was staring back at them and smiling slightly and shaking his head in disgust at the sight, and who was also, a minute later, taking *their* picture with the little yellow waterproof Minolta he'd brought with him.

The four viral musketeers, Rollin, Khan, Calain, and Le Guenno, now left the plane and walked toward the gate in the chain-link fence over by where some cars were parked. There were old cars, new cars, pickup trucks, vans, plus various scooters, motorcycles, and bikes. Some townspeople were there with their kids, billions of kids, plus some military types in maroon berets and olive drabs. There was a guy in the parking lot being interviewed by a video crew.

And then all of a sudden the journalists began to leave, the twenty journalists who'd come in on the same plane with the four scientists, they were piling their stuff and equipment into the cars and vans that had been standing by. Those cars had been waiting, it now became obvious, not for the scientists but for the *journalists,* who one by one were zooming out of Kikwit airport and heading off toward town.

The four heroes now looked around for something resembling an official welcoming committee. There didn't seem to be any. All that remained were some concrete buildings with scattered empty tables and chairs, the DC-3 being unloaded of its CDC cargo boxes, the village bystanders, and the man in the parking lot being interviewed by the video team.

Finally a guy drives up in a brand-new white Mercedes. From the looks of it, Bernard Le Guenno decides the car has not been sent to pick *them* up. The driver's in his twenties, sporty-looking, jaunty, with close-cropped hair, open white shirt, aviator-style sunglasses.

A Smilin' Jacques type of guy.

Le Guenno, who's brought his own little Canon videocam with him to Kikwit, now decides to pretend he's a journalist— it's the journalists, he's already concluded, who get the attention here—he decides to go over and interview this Smilin' Jacques character, just for the hell of it, while he's got nothing better to do.

"Are you waiting for someone?" Le Guenno asks the man, in English.

"I hardly understand English," says Smilin' Jacques in French.

"Do you want me to speak French?"

"Yes, it's better."

"What do you prefer, to receive the CDC team or the journalists?"

"Everybody, everybody."

"Is CNN very interesting for you?"

"Oh, yes, CNN is interesting because they do very good reporting."

"Is that going to stop the epidemic?"

"No, that's not going to stop the epidemic. Anyways . . ."

"Well, then, why do you want them to come?"

"To sensitize public opinion, world opinion."

"And the arrival of the experts, is that important for you?"

"Yes, I think it's important, and it reassures the population."

"Are you aware that they're supposed to come?"

"We're already aware that they have to come."

"You have information about the journalists but not about the experts?"

"No, we knew about the journalists but not about the experts."

"I see. And where do you get your news from?"

"From our radio . . . I mean . . . the diocese has a radio and this is how we knew about it. Every day, we get the news from Kinshasa."

"And the radio said nothing about the arrival of the experts?"

"Not the official radio, no."

"Thank you."

Le Guenno turned off his videocam.

The airport grasses waved in the breeze. The sun beat down on all their four heads. And Ali and Bernard and Philippe and Pierre stood there in the dust under the hot sun and gazed off toward the horizon and cursed the world and wondered what to do next, while the remaining villagers and the billion kids and Smilin' Jacques stood there and smiled politely and watched them.

That was their grand arrival into Kikwit.

5   Lady Bird Comes to CDC

The man in the parking lot turned out to be Tamfum Muyembe. Tamfum Muyembe was the Zairian virologist who'd been called to Kikwit to assess the hospital outbreak, had the blood samples taken from the dying patients, and sent them to Guido van der Groen in Antwerp. He was standing there in his pink shirt and dark pants, in front of a video team—cameraman, interviewer, and soundman, who was pointing a foot-long, foam-covered microphone at Muyembe, holding it out of camera range—talking steadily and at great length. This was now the main activity at Kikwit airport.

After an eternity they seemed to be finishing up, and so Bernard Le Guenno went over to Muyembe, tapped him on the shoulder, and said, "We're here." There was the usual round of greetings, backslapping, and inquiries after one's health. They loaded their bags and cargo into the van that Muyembe had driven up in, climbed in themselves, and at last the incoming medical saviors were driven away.

But not yet to the hospital. First stop was headquarters, located about a half mile from the hospital in a building that housed a private medical clinic. The clinic would serve as a base of operations for the scientists for the next three months. Here they got a briefing from David Heymann of the World Health Organization, which was the agency coordinating the international response to the crisis. Heymann had gotten there himself only two days previously. They also met Barbara Kierstiëns, of Médecins san Frontières (Doctors without Borders), of Brussels, who'd arrived in the city a day after Heymann.

So it was not until late in the afternoon, on toward evening, that Khan, Rollin, Calain, and Le Guenno got their first look at the hospital. The day had cooled down somewhat by that point, it was almost pleasant, when David Heymann drove them over. He took them past the cemetery, where there were a dozen or so new graves, all of them covered with fresh dirt. They were somewhat unnerving to Ali Khan: "You know, what you do as an epidemiologist is, you maintain these listings of people and their names and their age and sex and where they live and so on. But seeing their graves, all these freshly dug graves near the hospital, knowing that there were people buried under each of those wooden crosses—that brought a new meaning to the job. By the end of the outbreak I knew almost every name on those crosses."

And finally there was the hospital itself, a bunch of lonely blue buildings with corrugated tin roofs, spread out on a slight hill. To Ali Khan, the place looked dead and abandoned. "It was death. It was truly deserted," he said. "I mean it was empty. There were no health-care workers anywhere, nobody providing care for the patients. There were some family members outside, and there was a lot wailing going on amongst family members. It was pretty tragic."

They got out of the car and walked through the hospital grounds. There were ten separate pavilions connected by covered walkways. They went past the salle d'urgence (the emergency room), past the lab building, the pharmacy, the *salle d'opération* (the operating room). Garbage was strewn about here and there on the grass. Some goats were lying on the covered walkways, a dog.

And then they were at Pavilion 3, which housed the Ebola patients. There were open double doors leading into the pavilion, inside of which it was dark and quiet. The team members were still in their street clothes, the ones they'd arrived in, and they wore no protective equipment.

So they walked by the open doors, looked in, and went past.

From the start, the Communicable Disease Center had been part of the Public Health Service. As a branch of the federal government, the Public Health Service went back to 1798 when the nation's Fifth Congress passed, and president John Adams signed, "An Act for the Relief of Sick and Disabled Seamen." Seamen, as a result of their various activities on ship and shore, were subject to certain dangers and ailments, and this new act was designed to provide the sailors with proper hospitals and medical care. This medical care would not be free—the sailors were made to pay for it themselves, out of their own pockets, by a tax at the rate of twenty cents a month.

The first Marine Hospitals were built starting around 1800 in Boston, Norfolk, and New Orleans, all of which were seacoast cities and major ports. After a while, some other Marine Hospitals were going up at places not known for prime anchorage or proximity to the ocean, towns like Napoleon, Arkansas, and Paducah, Kentucky. The explanation was a matter of plain economics: a Marine Hospital meant lots of money to any area that could attract one. The program, after all, was known not as the Marine Hospital *Service* but rather as the Marine Hospital *Fund.* An 1855 U.S. Treasury Department report summarized the inevitable consequences: "In some towns there appears a desire to have Marine Hospitals so that additional sums of public money may there be expended. If this feeling not be checked, we shall have sinecure surgeons, sinecure stewards, sinecure matrons, sinecure nurses, without number. We have too many such already." In 1870, Wisconsin senator Thomas Howe underlined the point with the claim that "a favorite way of starting a town in the West, if it was anywhere on a stream or on a good-sized puddle, was to get an appropriation for a Marine Hospital."

The hospitals, indeed, started going up all over the country, but once finished they were not always well or intelligently used. The government addressed the problem straightforwardly by doing nothing at all, permitting the law of entropy to take effect. Between 1798 and 1869, thirty-one Marine Hospitals had been built at a total cost of $3 million, but by 1869 only nine of them were still functioning. Fourteen of the original thirty-one had been sold off for a combined sum of less than $400,000; others had been abandoned, one had burned down, and another had been washed into a river.

The solution, when it came, was to professionalize the health service by making it into a quasi-military organization and placing it under the control of a "surgeon general." There would be a Commissioned Corps of public health physicians, a band of health warriors who'd actually wear their own distinct uniforms. The Corps would constitute a professional elite, a separate class of government worker, one who was neither a political patronage appointee nor a soldier in the strict military sense, but rather something else in between. Their uniforms, supposedly, would mark out these people as an independent and autonomous team and express the notion of their working together in a common cause, united by a shared esprit de corps. By and large, these changes were effective, and they revolutionized the public health service.

The first uniforms were much in the railway-conductor mode, except that the letters *M.D.*, written in old-English script, appeared on each lapel. Later versions were designed on the

Navy model, which was why whenever the surgeon general appeared on television, be it C. Everett Koop or Joycelyn Elders, the viewer was left vaguely wondering, "Are they in the Navy Reserves, or what?"

From the beginning, the officers of the CDC's Epidemic Intelligence Service were required to wear their Commissioned Corps uniforms to work at least once a week, and on the mandatory day, which was Wednesday, people who'd showed up the day before in T-shirt, jeans, and Nikes would suddenly materialize in dress blues, summer whites, or all-purpose khakis according to season or mood or what they happened to have clean at the moment.

The freedom from political patronage allegedly enjoyed by regular members of the Commissioned Corps did not extend to the directors of the Centers for Disease Control, who were customarily relieved of command by the incoming presidential administration. Since the agency's inception in 1946 there had been more than a dozen CDC chiefs, directors, or acting heads, some of whom were in office for as little as a year or two before being removed in a wave of political housecleaning. One chief, David Sencer, was fired on national television by Joseph Califano, Jimmy Carter's secretary of health, education, and welfare, who, as the cameras rolled, looked Sencer in the eye and said, "I want to say something nice about you: 'Even though Dr. Sencer is not going to be with us anymore, we appreciate his contributions.' "

Sencer got home that night just in time to watch the nightly news and see himself get fired on television. But who could blame Joe Califano? He was only looking for "some fresh air, some fresh faces" at the CDC, as he explained the next day.

The strongly provisional nature of the CDC's top job made the post into something less than a plum, and no Nobel Prize winners or other scientists of equal caliber had been known to apply for the post. The National Institutes of Health, by contrast, was presided over in the mid-1990s by Harold Varmus, recipient of the 1989 Nobel Prize in physiology or medicine for his work on oncogenes.

James L. Goddard, the first chief to take office in the CDC's new headquarters building, absolutely never wanted to be head of the Communicable Disease Center. So much did he detest the job that when informed of the appointment by his boss, Assistant Surgeon General Arnold Kurlander, who had selected him, Goddard's first words to Kurlander were "You bastard!"

Goddard, who was on record as actually preferring the directorship of the godforsaken Indian Health Service to being made CDC chief, only accepted the position because he viewed it as a stepping-stone to much greater things, like a surgeon generalship. Still, Goddard made the best of a bad situation and responded by making the CDC into his own private fiefdom. He wore his uniform to work every day of the week, required his subordinates to wear theirs at any and all official functions, and brought in Army bands to play military marches at awards ceremonies.

But there were even loftier rewards than that to being made head of the Communicable Disease Center, for the holder of that majestic position had now reached "flag rank," meaning that he got to fly his personal "star flag" on the pole in front of Building 1, the six-story administration building at 1600 Clifton Road.

There were actually *two* flags: a yellow one for when the director was away from the office and a separate white pennant for when he was actually there, on board and in command, striding the decks, captain of the Good Ship Disease Control.

It was not the CDC's policy to import new diseases into the country. The whole point of the place was to *curtail* infectious outbreaks, not to expand them: its famed EIS officers went out into the wilds where they halted an epidemic in its tracks, after which the roving disease commandos came back to Atlanta until the next crisis arose. But in 1969, about a year before the CDC's eradication teams had made West Africa smallpox-free, a respected and experienced CDC physician brought a hitherto unknown viral disease onto U.S. shores for the first time.

Like many another case of viral hemorrhagic fever, this one first appeared in a hospital setting, in the Church of the Brethren Mission clinic in Lassa, Nigeria, when on a Sunday morning in January 1969, Laura Wine, a mission nurse in her late sixties, came down with some mild back pain and generalized weakness. Nothing all that unusual, but soon enough this had escalated to a high fever and a sore throat so painful that even swallowing liquids was almost impossible. Her condition failed to respond to penicillin and streptomycin, both of which were antibiotics, which was a telltale sign that a virus of some sort was at work. Nevertheless, the symptoms did not precisely fit any viral disease that her attending physician, Dr. John Hamer, was familiar with, and so he had Laura Wine flown out of Lassa to the city of Jos, where there was a properly equipped, relatively sophisticated medical institution, the Bingham Memorial Hospital. There, Laura Wine was cared for by an American nurse by the name of Charlotte Shaw.

On the same day that Laura Wine was admitted, Charlotte Shaw had accidentally pricked a finger while she was picking roses from her flower garden. She treated the wound and forgot about it, but later on, while swabbing out Laura Wine's throat, Charlotte Shaw felt a distinct stinging sensation in the finger she'd cut earlier, and which was now protected only by a thin gauze wrapping, no gloves. Laura Wine's condition, meanwhile, had deteriorated; she was bleeding from bodily orifices and from needle puncture sites, and within thirty hours of her admittance to Bingham Memorial Hospital, she died.

Eight days later, Charlotte Shaw herself fell ill with a backache, headache, and leg pains, followed by chills and then a fever that topped out at 104.8°. Small red rashes appeared on her face, neck, and arms, then spread out to the rest of her body. Strange ulcers broke out in her throat. Her skin turned blue. And on the eleventh day of her illness, she died.

Jeanette Troup, the hospital's only full-time physician, performed an autopsy on Charlotte Shaw; Lily "Penny" Pinneo, a Johns Hopkins–trained Presbyterian nurse, assisted at the operating table. They found large quantities of yellowish serum pooling up inside Charlotte Shaw's body, a residue of internal hemorrhaging. They found diseased kidneys, a clogged heart, lungs unnaturally red with blood, and a liver plugged up by dead cells and fat deposits. During the postmortem, both Pinneo and Troup wore gowns and gloves, but on the theory that they couldn't any longer infect the patient, who was already dead, neither of them wore face masks.

Two weeks later Penny Pinneo, in turn, fell ill with the same signs and symptoms, at which point the CDC entered the picture.

Lyle Conrad was the CDC's number one disaster-relief officer in Lagos, Nigeria. He was a big man with glasses and beard, another in the long line of CDC disease-fighters who'd started out as normal doctors but soon grew to hate the ordinary practice of medicine. In the United States, a conventional medical practice meant dealing day in and day out with the same predictable and boring complaints, people with back pains, bunions, bad colds, and heart problems. "To me it was totally uninteresting," he said. "Taking care of chronic cardiac patients the rest of my life, the overweight, the obese—it was just not exciting."

Tropical medicine *was*, however, as he'd learned early on at Northwestern University where as an undergrad research assistant for a malariologist he worked with a range of weird diseases such as chicken malaria and hemogregorin parasites in snakes. One summer he'd had to examine all the snakes in the Chicago Zoo for signs of hemogregorin bacteria. They'd be delivered to the lab in boxes and he'd have fifteen or twenty snakes coiling up and stretching themselves out and crawling around in there, and he'd take blood from them and map out all their parasites, and he loved it.

And so a year or two after getting out of George Washington University medical school, he was in Enugu, Nigeria, where he faced down three major epidemics in a row: smallpox, measles, and meningococcal meningitis, the latter of which had killed about ten thousand children. During the measles outbreak he worked with three Nigerian doctors at a pediatrics clinic in Lagos, and they saw a thousand patients per day for six weeks.

"We'd come to work every morning and each of us would see two hundred to two hundred and fifty cases of just plain measles in these kids for about six weeks' time. There was no room at the hospital for a thousand kids a day, so you did the best you could on an outpatient basis."

Measles was a killer if it turned into pneumonia, which it often did, but all he could do was to treat the kids in the examining room—put them on antibiotics, hook them up temporarily to an IV drip in the hospital if they were severely dehydrated—and send them back out again. The experience convinced him that the only effective way of handling such disasters was by preventing them from happening in the first place. That meant public health, of course, treating people en masse, in huge collectivities, instead of just one by one in the doctor's office. This was the outlook that had brought him to the CDC in 1965, and it was where he'd remain for the rest of his professional life.

He was on his way back to Atlanta in March 1969 when he got a call from Stan Foster, the CDC's smallpox-eradication specialist in the Lagos area. A nurse by the name of Penny Pinneo, Foster told Conrad, was in Lagos waiting to be shipped out to New York. Nobody knew what was wrong with her, nobody could get her aboard a commercial flight, and could he help? The Lagos University Hospital had refused to admit the patient, he said, who was at that point stretched out in the

Pest House, a hot and hellacious tin-roofed shed that had been used as an isolation ward for smallpox patients.

Next morning, Lyle Conrad drove over to the Pest House, which at that point seemed to be populated with every CDC person in the immediate vicinity: Conrad himself, Stan Foster, Karl Western, and Herman Gray, all four of them members of the Epidemic Intelligence Service. With twenty years' worth of tropical medicine experience among them, the four M.D.s now examined Penny Pinneo.

"She was obtunded—flaked out, no energy," Conrad recalled years later. "She could hardly talk, she was so weak. She was low-grade fever, she was absolutely flat. She could hardly sit up. She kept passing out every time we lifted her head up, it was amazing. She hadn't had anything to eat, she'd had nausea, vomiting. Her chief complaint, though, was a bitching sore throat."

This was some weird new disease, Conrad thought.

"We've got to get her out of here," he said to Stan Foster. "I'm going back home in two days. If you can keep her alive until Monday, I'll take her back with me . . . but how do we get her past immigration?"

"Well, that's easy," said Stan Foster. "After all, she hasn't got any quarantinable disease, right?"

That much was true: if this was a new disease, then it wouldn't show up on any quarantine lists. So the four of them crafted a letter to the U.S. Foreign Quarantine Service, a carefully worded document stating that although Penny Pinneo wasn't exactly the picture of health, she nevertheless had no quarantinable disease. They also stated that although she had an infectious condition—the Laura Wine, Charlotte Shaw, Penny Pinneo pattern had established that fact decisively—she was nevertheless not at that point infectious.

Inasmuch as this was a new disease that none of them had ever seen before, the question arises how they could have known this.

"Well, we went through every virus disease that we could think of," said Conrad, "and how many virus diseases do you know of that are still infectious after two or three weeks? As a category, most virus diseases are infectious right before they come on and for the first few days afterwards, and then they go into this latent phase. She had been sick for fourteen to twenty-one days."

And how did they know it was a *viral* disease?

"We were pretty sure it was," he said. "We thought it was an arbovirus. It didn't look like any bacterial disease that we'd seen, and we had categorized it as an arboviral disease of some kind."

And so Monday, March 3, 1969, two Nigerian orderlies carried Penny Pinneo onto a Pan American Airways Boeing 707 passenger jet and strapped her into a draped-off area in the first-class section. The first two rows on the left-hand side had been removed, and the area had been converted into an intensive-care unit.

Lyle Conrad sat just across the aisle. On the floor to his right, in a little portable cooler filled with ice cubes, were the last mortal remains of the first two victims of Lassa fever: various blood, brain, liver, and kidney sections of Laura Wine and Charlotte Shaw. Sitting in the window seat beside Conrad was Dorothy Davis, the nurse who had taken care of Pinneo in the Pest House, and who was now close to exhaustion.

Conrad was busy the entire flight. Because of her inability to swallow, Pinneo's throat kept piling up fluids that had to be sucked out every so often, which Conrad did with a bulb syringe, a turkey-baster sort of apparatus, which he emptied out into a kidney basin, which he then got rid of in the plane's toilet. He also refreshed the ice in the specimen cooler, pouring off the melt into the lavatory sink and then refilling the cooler with new ice from the ship's galley.

The plane stopped in Accra, Ghana; Monrovia, Liberia; and Dakar, Senegal, taking on new passengers at each point, then flew nonstop to New York. The whole trip took about eighteen hours.

At Kennedy Airport, the passengers got off, then Conrad came down the stairs bringing the cooler with him, and finally Penny Pinneo was carried down on the stretcher. The prepared letter worked perfectly, the customs and immigration people had no problem with any of it, and Lassa fever was thereby brought into the United States.

David J. Sencer, chief of the CDC, was not ecstatic about Lyle Conrad's bringing Penny Pinneo into the country with a new viral hemorrhagic fever.

"What do you mean bringing back missionaries from overseas with dangerous infectious diseases?" he yelled. "That is not CDC's business! Did you ever think of how you were endangering people on that airplane?"

"He railed at me for half an hour," Lyle Conrad recalled later. But Conrad had been prepared for this and had his ducks in a row.

"Absolutely, we very carefully thought about that," Conrad told Sencer. "In fact, I've got the whole passenger manifest. But until me and the nurse get sick, you don't have to worry about the people on the airplane: we were the ones most intimately involved with her. Pinneo's fourteen to twenty-one days into whatever illness it is, so she's not very infectious. Anyway she doesn't have any quarantinable disease. But even if she did, sick Americans anywhere in the world are entitled to come back to their own country for decent medical care—or to die here, if it comes to that."

But it made no difference to Dave Sencer, who pulled Conrad off the Pinneo case.

Penny Pinneo eventually recovered from Lassa fever, although it took about three months. Neither Conrad nor Dorothy Davis, Pinneo's nurse, nor anyone else on the plane from

Africa, so far as was known, ever contracted the disease, and in later years even Dave Sencer changed his mind about Conrad's bringing Pinneo back to the country: "I think it was probably a damn good thing that he brought her back," he said much later. "We learned what causes Lassa fever and how to diagnose it, we learned how to manage cases in terms of hospital precautions and so on. If he hadn't brought the nurse back, we might still be in the dark about the disease. So retrospectively I give him a big pat on the back for it."

Still, viruses had a habit of spreading like viruses. They were small and invisible, you couldn't see them coming or going, and it was hard to keep them bottled up. And so within three months of its importation, Lassa fever broke out in the United States, first in Connecticut and then in Pennsylvania, where it killed one person. The new cases, however, hadn't come from direct contact with Penny Pinneo: they'd come from the laboratory, from the Lassa samples in vials and in cell cultures. The pathogen had escaped from the sample bottles, something that viruses were exceptionally skilled at doing.

The laboratory in question was Yale University's Arbovirus Research Unit, which was run by Jordi Casals, a world-renowned and highly experienced virologist. He and his colleagues had been running the Lassa specimens through various tests in an attempt to identify the infectious agent. They'd tested it against two hundred different types of virus reagents and never got a match, supporting Conrad's view that this was indeed a new viral disease. But then on June 3, 1969, exactly three months after Lassa fever arrived in New York, Casals himself fell ill with the virus, this despite his having regularly protected himself by means of goggles, mask, and gloves.

Since there was no known cure, he was injected with some of Penny Pinneo's blood plasma on the theory that since she'd survived the disease, her serum must harbor the antibodies that had neutralized the virus and saved her life. If they worked for her, they ought to work for him, too. That, anyway, was the theory; valid or not, Jordi Casals survived Lassa fever.

Keeping Lassa samples around in the laboratory, however, was proving to be an extremely dangerous proposition. Sonja Buckley, who worked in the Yale lab, did *not* always use a face mask when working with the virus, and in fact she even made a practice of "mouth pipetting" sample liquids.

A pipette was an open glass tube—it looked much like a soda straw—that had volumetric graduation marks etched along the side. You dipped one end in the solution, placed the other end in your mouth, and drew up a given quantity of the liquid, exactly as if you were sipping a mint julep. Back then, this was standard practice, it was normal procedure in biological laboratories. To "protect" yourself against accidental ingestion of some highly dangerous liquid, you might go so far as to stuff a bit of cotton in the upper end of the pipette (as if that would stop any self-respecting viral agent).

Naive as it appeared in hindsight, the system seemed to work, and for unknown reasons lab personnel did not drop dead right and left. Still, many near-disasters occurred, and one time when Sonja Buckley was about to draw up some of Penny Pinneo's infected serum, the pipette proved to be just a bit too short to reach the sample. So Buckley tilted the bottle back so that the serum would creep up forward along the side of the bottle, she tilted it back, and back, and back . . . until the open bottle top was touching the tip of her nose.

"It was a stupid thing to do," she said years later. "Utterly stupid."

But Sonia Buckley never even got sick.

Juan Ramon did get sick, however, and he didn't even work with Lassa virus. He worked down the hall from Jordi Casals and Sonja Buckley, on Eastern equine encephalitis, and so far as anyone knew, he'd never even been near the Lassa samples. But late in November, six months after the lab got the first Lassa specimens, he came down with a case of something or other: fever, chills, muscle pains, et cetera—nobody knew what it was. A clinic doctor took a sample of Juan Ramon's blood and sent to a commercial lab for analysis while Ramon went home to York, Pennsylvania, for Thanksgiving.

Ten days after his first symptoms, Juan Ramon died. Tests showed he died from Lassa fever.

The commercial lab now incinerated all of Juan Ramon's blood, and Yale University terminated its Lassa work. The *New York Times* ran a story about the incident, headlining it: "New fever virus so deadly that research halts."

Yale University wanted nothing further to do with Lassa fever or the virus that caused it, and so Jordi Casals collected together all the Lassa samples, packaged them up, and sent them to the Communicable Disease Center in Atlanta.

There, at least, they knew how to keep viruses in the bottle.

Viruses were so small that they were composed of countable numbers of atoms: you could look at them in an electron microscope and actually see the distinct molecular groupings that they were made up of. By the adroit use of DNA sequencing machines and the other tools of molecular biology, you could also read out a given virus's genome, the complete set of nucleotide sequences that constituted its molecular identity.

Despite a size near the vanishing point, viruses had been discovered a long time ago, back before the turn of the century, by two European botanists working independently on tobacco mosaic disease. Tobacco was a major cash crop, and the disease, which appeared as a mosaic-like mottling on tobacco leaves, was interfering with production and causing financial losses.

First to investigate the matter was the Russian botanist Dimitri Ivanovsky, who got interested in the problem while a student at St. Petersburg University in 1890, the year a tobacco mosaic epidemic ripped across the plantations of the Crimea.

The disease was thought to be spread by bacteria, which at the time was an entirely logical assumption. Some twenty-five years earlier, in 1865, Pasteur had definitively established the germ theory of disease, according to which illnesses were caused by tiny organisms, bacteria, which were passed from one individual to the next. Bacteria could infect plants, too, and so it was a reasonable inference that they had caused the tobacco mottling.

Ivanovsky aimed to isolate the microbe responsible, and so in 1892 he crushed a quantity of tobacco leaves and passed the juice through a so-called Chamberland candle, a type of filter that had been invented by Pasteur's assistant Charles Chamberland in 1884. This long, thin wick inside of a glass tube was white and looked like a candle, but in fact it was a fine-screen porcelain filtration column. You poured in a liquid at the top and anything that came out at the bottom was extremely clean and free of impurities, including bacteria, which were collected out at the top.

But when Ivanovsky passed the sap from diseased tobacco plants through a Chamberland candle, the purified liquid still caused the disease when he rubbed it on the leaves of healthy plants. This was anomalous: the bacteria that he'd seen through the microscope beforehand were no longer visible in the liquid that had passed through the filter, but the filtered liquid was capable of causing the disease just as it had at the outset. The disease, therefore, had to be a product of something other than ordinary bacteria.

Six years later, in 1898, Martinus Beijerinck, a Dutch botanist working at the Delft Polytechnic School, repeated Ivanovsky's experiments and got the same results: the sap from tobacco mosaic leaves was just as infectious after the filtration as it had been earlier. The pathogen, whatever it was, couldn't be bacterial, he decided, because it refused to grow in a normal culture medium outside the plant, whereas most bacteria grew there like wildfire. Nor was the agent a toxin, a liquid poison, because the filtered tobacco juice caused a chain infection in a series of plants, the sap from one plant infecting the next one in sequence, which meant that the pathogen was indeed multiplying inside the plants, a feat that an inert poison wouldn't be capable of.

The infectious agent, he reasoned, must be a living thing because it grew and multiplied, but it couldn't be a bacterium because it couldn't be cultured in the conventional manner. Beijerinck therefore concluded that he was dealing with a completely new type of life-form, a *contagium vivum fluidum*, a contagious living fluid. He also coined the term *filterable virus*, *virus* being the Latin for poison. This new entity, he said, did not have the power of reproducing itself directly, but multiplied itself only inside living cells: "The contagium, in order to reproduce, must be incorporated into the living protoplasm of the cell, into whose reproduction it is, in a manner of speaking, passively drawn." The statement was prophetic, for it exactly described how viruses operated, by inserting themselves into cells where they got multiplied repeatedly, the details of which weren't fully worked out till much later.

Other researchers were soon finding new viruses, and in 1898, the German scientists Friedrich Löffler and Paul Frosch discovered that foot-and-mouth disease, which affected cattle, was caused by a virus. And in 1900 the American military surgeon Walter Reed showed that a virus was the cause of yellow fever, a mosquito-borne hemorrhagic disease prevalent in the tropics.

It gradually became apparent what sort of a miracle machine a virus really was. It escaped almost all the normal requirements for life: it had no metabolic machinery of its own, took in no food, and gave off no waste products, whether in the form of heat, light, or any other form of matter or energy. Nevertheless, it managed to self-replicate, a feat that it performed by exporting off to other entities all the processes that could be carried on elsewhere while retaining for itself only what was inseparable from its personal identity, namely its distinct genetic makeup. Somehow, viruses had stripped themselves down to the minimum allowance of what was required for life, then stripped themselves down still further, until they possessed *less* than the minimum requirement, borrowing from host cells the extra stuff necessary for reproduction.

You really had to hand it to these viruses: they were damned crafty entities. They weren't even alive, much less conscious, but yet they had solved the central problem of existence: they forced more complicated organisms to do their dirty work for them, while they themselves just sat back and relaxed and got propagated.

Who could fail to admire those tiny marvels? Viruses were so very clever, so extremely ingenious in the way they operated and perpetuated themselves, that it was almost an honor to be infected by them.

Almost.

In the end, wiping out the smallpox virus in ten years really was an overambitious hope. It took eleven years. It took from 1966 to 1977, the year of the world's last case of naturally occurring smallpox. The patient was a twenty-three-year-old Somali cook named Ali Maalin, a tall, thin man who survived the disease and became briefly famous as the last in a long line of cases that stretched way back into the prehistory of infectious diseases.

Then, one by one, the world's nations were certified to be smallpox free by the World Health Organization. Freedom from smallpox had to be established by physical proof, by taking blood samples from suspect cases and testing them in the laboratory, and many of the tests were done at the CDC. During 1978, the CDC's smallpox lab reviewed more than four thousand samples for the virus, every last one of which proved negative. On December 9, 1979, therefore, in Geneva, twenty members of the WHO smallpox eradication team signed a parchment that said simply: "We, the members of the global commission for the certification of smallpox eradication, certify that smallpox has been eradicated from the world."

The main obstacles to eradication, it turned out, had not been scientific or medical but rather social: for reasons of their own, whether out of religion, superstition, or plain fear, some people just didn't want to be vaccinated. But universal vaccination had not proved necessary, and the disease had been eradicated without it.

So smallpox was now history, the first virus deliberately made extinct through human design and intention. You could read about smallpox in history books. You could go to the library and read accounts of how the Egyptian ruler Ramses V, who died in 1157 B.C., had suffered from it. You could even see pictures of his mummified head, with the pockmarks on his face clearly visible to the naked eye.

What you could not do any longer was go out to the wild and see an actual living case of the disease, anywhere in the world. There *were* no more cases: the virus, every last particle of it, had been entirely removed from the natural order.

It was gone.

Despite its being home to the rarest diseases, the worst viruses, the deadliest pathogens, the CDC was the ultimate self-amplifying federal bureaucracy—and how could it not be? After all, who could object to any institutional excess, any expenditure or innovative new program, so long as it was done in the name of "health"? And so the place was always building itself up, expanding, and heading off in important new directions. Every new chief, as if to justify his existence, ordered new management survey assessment initiatives, mind-pulverizing nomenclature adjustments, tectonic shifts in the extant institutional alignments and arrangements, all of which were absolutely unintelligible to the outside world.

The CDC was forever being "reorganized." This was apparently so crucial to an incoming director's sense of self and inner worth that directors couldn't keep themselves from "reorganizing" the place even if they wanted to.

Divisions became *branches* and *branches* became *bureaus.* *Units* became *programs* and *programs* became *centers.* *Centers* were subdivided into *divisions,* which were subdivided into *branches.* The CDC itself, once merely a *bureau,* became an *agency.* *Chiefs* became *directors.* Consequential new acronyms were invented: the Division of Industrial Hygiene (DIH) became the Bureau of Occupational Safety and Health (BOSH).

The place itself never had the same name for more than a few years running. Malaria Control in War Areas became the Communicable Disease Center became the National Communicable Disease Center became the Center for Disease Control became the Centers for Disease Control became the Centers for Disease Control and Prevention. Nevertheless, except when it was, for the space of three fleeting years, the NCDC, it was always the CDC, even when, by rights and strictly speaking, it should have been the CDCP. But that was the way of government bureaucracy, and nobody really paid much attention to it all.

Lady Bird Johnson came down to the CDC one time—this was in 1964, when it was still the Communicable Disease Center—for a little half-day tour of the place. Naturally, this was an opportunity that could not go officially unrecognized, and so a bit of a groundbreaking ceremony was arranged inasmuch as a new $12-million building happened to be going up on the premises. Nothing special, just your ordinary $12-million auditorium. Two silver shovels were ordered for the occasion— only the best for the first lady!—to be wielded by Lady Bird herself and the current chief, James Goddard.

The day of the ceremony, administrators gave speeches, military brass from the three services looked on, Goddard officiated in his dress whites while his personal "star flag" snapped in the breeze high above the Good Ship Disease Control, and Lady Bird herself shoveled the first spadeful of dirt.

That is, she tried to. The ground was rock hard at the site of her first attempt, and so she moved over a few inches and tried again. With no better luck.

This went on for a while, the first lady pecking around at the ground like a chicken. Meanwhile Bob Shakleford, the official groundskeeper, was looking all over for the parcel of dirt that he'd prepared in advance. He'd dug a hole and filled it with soft peat moss, then covered it back over again with regular dirt, leveling it off and making it indistinguishable from the rest. It was so well disguised that even he couldn't find it again.

Without warning, Lady Bird now approached the spot in question, jabbed her shovel in, really leaned into it, and the ground was so soft that she lurched headlong . . . *whoops!* . . . nearly falling right in.

Lady Bird's husband, Lyndon Baines Johnson, architect of "the Great Society," decided in 1965 that great societies did not include rats in inner-city neighborhoods, and so a rat control bill was forwarded to Congress. This was an immediate hit with the congressmen, who entertained the proposed legislation with all the appropriate gravity. Why, they wanted to know, were only *city* rats being targeted? Were country rats being discriminated against? There were snide comments about "four-legged rats" versus "two-legged rats." One member of Congress, clearly not an admirer of the bill, said that "the rat smart thing to do" would be to vote the bill down "rat now."

Nevertheless, a Rat Control Act was passed together with a $40-million appropriation for the first two years of the program, and the CDC soon found itself presiding over some of the nation's finest moments in rat control. It gave rat control courses; it hired seventy new people; and in the words of Elizabeth Etheridge, the CDC's official historian, "Many unskilled people got entry-level jobs looking for rat holes." ("Except for affecting the stress level," she added, "it had nothing to do with health.")

At the other extreme, the CDC also went into space, protecting civilization from "moon germs." Director Jim Goddard was behind the idea, and he created the Interagency Committee on Back Contamination to deal with the threat. Returning astronauts were to be quarantined for three weeks, even though, prior to being isolated, they'd be bobbing around on the high seas in open air after having emerged from the spacecraft. The plan was that biological isolation garments would be thrown to the astros through the open hatch, they'd put the garments on, then spray each other off with great quantities of iodine solution and household bleach.

"No lunar bugs can survive such a bath, we like to believe," said astronaut Michael Collins. "Although what prevents them from escaping into the sea I don't really know."

CDC lab people inspected moon rocks for germs and other extraterrestrial creatures. "I'll never forget that when they started inoculating some of the ground-up moon dust into conventional tissue culture, everything died," said Walter Dowdle, chief of the CDC virology section. "Of course everything died. When you put dirt in tissue culture, it dies.

"I never felt so silly in my life," he added.

Later, when the CDC got still another new director and was therefore put through yet one more of its perennial self-assessment studies—the basis, of course, for "a complete reorganization"—a committee of sixteen outside experts, the so-called Red Book Committee, was asked to put together a list of the nation's ten most pressing health problems. It was to be a roster of major public health threats, clear and present dangers to the citizenry of the United States.

Almost making the cut—number twelve on the list, finally dropped off only after much heated debate—was . . . hernia.

Hernia!

6 The Lab of Last Resort

Standing there in the center aisle of Pavilion 3, Pierre Rollin was surrounded by the dead and dying.

"It was very bad," he said. "People were vomiting; there was diarrhea and blood all over the floors and walls. The dead were lying among the living."

"There were these metals beds with mattresses, no sheets, people dying on the mattresses," said Ali Khan. "This long corridor split in half . . . there were two dead people lying there who nobody had moved. It was horrible. I mean just a whole bunch of people dying of Ebola hemorrhagic fever. And there was nothing you could do for them."

"We had a quick look inside," Philippe Calain said. "It was impressive. But the light was not good, and when we came back the same afternoon, it was much more impressive than what we had thought. Because then you could see the cadavers that you didn't really see before, because they were covered.

101

You saw the patients closer, you could see what the needle hazard was—there were needles everywhere: on the floor, in the beds, in plastic bags in the nurses' room."

The room was cramped, claustrophobic, and reeked of death. The floors were slippery with blood, vomit, human excrement, urine, dried pools of unknown stuff. One patient's bowels had emptied out on the mattress; the patient slipped down off the bed and onto the floor, where he lay curled up in fetal position, emaciated and naked, crabbed and bent like a dead sparrow.

On the other side of the building there was another ward, a mirror image of the first, except that it held no living patients.

"There were two or three cadavers there," said Philippe Calain, "some of them I think for three days."

Off in a separate area, across a grassy court toward the rear of the hospital complex, was Pavilion 9. Pavilion 9 was a small white stucco building that at one time had been used to house children who had measles. From the outside, it looked almost pleasant: it had a covered porch with a couple of wooden benches that faced out toward the grass, and you could imagine yourself sitting there in the shade and enjoying a drink. Now it held three adults.

"There was a corpse and two people," said Bernard Le Guenno. "It was a mother and the daughter, lying in the same bed. They had been there for three days alone."

"They were completely alone," said Philippe Calain. "One was already dead for sure, one was alive, the other one was moribund. We didn't know what to do, there are so many things to do, so we just left them like that."

The following morning, the mother was dead, the daughter still alive beside her mother's corpse, the two of them side by side on the same narrow mattress. "We had a better way to help now," said Calain, "and we took this lady, still alive, to Pavilion 3. She died later, but maybe in not so terrible conditions."

"It was very risky to have needle sticks," said Pierre Rollin, "so we tried to limit the number of perfusions, the number of injections. When we found that a patient developed the very bad symptoms—fast breathing, hiccups, bleeding—we tried to get them rested, to calm them, so they didn't feel anxious or whatever. But you don't try very fancy intensive-care things because there's no way that you're going to cure them."

There were no cures for these people, no treatments, drugs, or proven therapies for Ebola, and so there was no way of controlling the course of the disease once the virus started replicating itself and eating away at the insides of the victim. Over and above the physical pain it caused, there was a separate sense of terror and fear, the victim's realization that what was happening to his life and body was now beyond the power of medicine to influence or arrest. For the patient, matters were out of control in the most absolute and total sense: nothing the patient did, nothing the doctor could do, would make any difference to the final outcome. The victim's fate had been sealed well in advance, and events would now proceed of their own course while the patient lay there and waited and watched.

The doctors talked to their patients and listened to them.

"Most of the time they said they were thirsty," said Calain. "Not mainly because they had nothing to drink, but because one of the symptoms of the disease is a very sore throat and pain in swallowing. That was one of their main complaints— that and extreme weakness, weakness that you suffer of. It's difficult to imagine lying on a bed and suffering from being weak. Even lifting their head was a big, huge effort."

"They all were very tired," said Pierre Rollin. "Some say that they had headache, chest pain, back pain. Most of them don't want to talk, they're too exhausted to talk. They don't want to do anything, they just want to die. That's one of the signs of Ebola: people are really very exhausted, the *whole* time.

"They ask for water—treat me, do me something—they ask to die with the family around."

The dying patients had a uniform appearance: they had a fixed stare, gazing upward, their face a mask, ghostlike and expressionless.

"At the end of the disease," said Calain, "the patient does not look, from the outside, as horrible as you can read in some books: they are not 'melting,' they are not full of blood. They're in shock, muscular shock. They are not unconscious, but you would say 'obtunded'—dull, quiet, very tired."

"Very few were hemorrhaging, hemorrhage is not the main symptom," said Rollin. "Less than half of the patients had some kind of hemorrhage. But the ones that bled, died."

"So many people died," said Philippe Calain. "And so many people died in difficult conditions. We were helpful, but not as much as we would have wished. We stopped the transmission among health-care workers, and we made the patients feel that they were no longer abandoned. That was something, even if we couldn't cure them."

The cleanup took five days. Pierre Rollin and Philippe Calain were the ones who did it, were the ones who actually went inside Pavilion 3, turned it back into a hospital ward, and reclaimed it for the practice of medicine.

"One of the problems that we found there was that everybody was afraid to go into the ward and take care of the patients," Pierre Rollin said later. "That's why we found dead people—the people who were dead for two or three days—because nobody wanted to do anything. So what we did—it was mostly Philippe Calain and myself—we just went in, cleaned the floor, removed the needles, removed the cadavers, put them in body bags, did the cleaning."

The needles. The preferred method for drug delivery in African hospitals was by injection: that way a doctor could be sure the patient got the proper dose of the drug in question, there was no fumbling around with pills, for the taking of which drinking water was sometimes not available. Often the doctor or nurse just dropped the syringe and left it where it lay, and so there were used needles all over Pavilion 3. They crunched and popped underfoot as you walked.

"The first thing I did the first day was to really hunt the needles, every place possible, and we found a lot," said Calain. "This was the first thing to do, I think, and you can realize that in this condition you don't have much time to take care of the patients. But I think that was the emergency on this very first day."

He and Rollin would get there early in the morning, suit up in plastic gowns, aprons, face masks, and goggles, then they'd walk through a pool of bleach and make their entry into the pavilion. There they'd find new corpses, excrement, blood, and stench. They'd spray the cadavers with bleach, put them into body bags, spray them again, put them on stretchers or the gurney, and get them out of the hospital ward.

They disinfected any and all contaminated surfaces, which in this case meant most of the ward and everything in it. They scraped up vomit, urine, and excreta off the floors, put it into buckets, then emptied the buckets into a prepared ditch. They swabbed the place down with mops, then disinfected surfaces with power sprayers, spraying the floors, walls, beds, and mattresses with bleach, of which they had three different concentrations: the strongest for the cadavers, blood, and human waste, a weaker solution for beds and walls, and the weakest of all for the skin of a living patient.

They trained new hospital workers at Bandundu University, a medical college a few blocks away, brought them to the hospital, and took them into the pavilion where they helped with the cleanup and with patient care. Pierre and Philippe often worked the whole day through and into the night, sometimes staying on in the pavilion till midnight. After sundown, which occurred about six o'clock, there'd be some artificial lighting when the gasoline-powered generators were working, but gasoline wasn't always available for the generators, so they'd work with headlights strapped to their heads or with flashlights or by the light of kerosene lamps.

Later, in the morgue, a separate building over by Pavilion 9, Pierre Rollin and sometimes Ali Khan would take biopsies of the dead, "especially the ones whose evolution was not clear," said Rollin. "We had some people who came in the ward and died in the following hours without any way to have a physical exam on them. So we took a small sample of the liver to get confirmatory diagnosis."

A needle biopsy was straightforward enough in ordinary circumstances. You used a large-bore needle that you forced through the skin; you pushed a plunger that clipped off some tissue, then you released the plunger and withdrew the needle and sample. It was not an especially safe procedure to perform on a newly dead Ebola patient, but the CDC doctors did them anyway, sometimes on patients whose names they didn't even know.

"One case, all we knew was this woman had been left by her family—deserted at the doorstep by some family members," said Ali Khan. "Not sure who she was. She had the clinical disease and hemorrhage and she died the next morning. And so we did the biopsy on her."

That was the routine, every day for five days, after which Calain and Rollin had created a hospital ward that was clean, neat, and orderly. Each patient had his own bed. There were plastic covers on the mattresses. The walls and floors were washed and dry. Basic sanitary procedures had been set up. Fresh water was available.

Not a single used needle was anywhere in sight.

The weird part of the Kikwit crisis was the way it seemed to be a video replay of another Ebola epidemic in another Zairian hospital nearly twenty years earlier.

"The funny thing is, my former boss went to Zaire in '76 for an outbreak of Ebola, and he was cleaning the floor and taking care of nurses who got Ebola and died, and twenty years after I've been to the same country and have done exactly the same thing," said Pierre Rollin. "Amazing, to be doing the same thing twenty years later."

In 1976, in the town of Yambuku in the northern part of Zaire, people were dying en masse in a small village hospital staffed by Catholic nuns. It was a scene of nurses and used needles, of samples being flown to Antwerp, of a Kinshasa-based American doctor calling the CDC for assistance, of families preparing victims for burial and then contracting the disease themselves, of people fleeing the hospital in terror for their lives. Indeed, the worst of it was that in both cases the hospital itself was the focal point, host, and main amplifier of the epidemic.

Yambuku was a village in the tropical rain forests north of the river Congo. Although it lacked a doctor and was staffed only by relatively untrained Catholic nuns, nurses, and midwives, the Yambuku Mission Hospital was the primary source of health care for the sixty thousand people who lived in the Yandongi collectivity, one of seven counties that made up the Bumba Zone. The hospital was a collection of tin-roofed concrete pavilions housing a pharmacy, operating room, and a total of 120 beds. It was about one-third the size of Kikwit General Hospital, which it also resembled in having no electricity and a shortage of basic medical supplies and equipment.

The mission hospital, nonetheless, ran an outpatient clinic that handled as many as four hundred patients a day. People would come in with everything from malaria to dysentery to filariasis, a mosquito-borne disease that caused a person's legs to swell up almost to the size of an elephant's leg. Whatever the ailment, treatment usually consisted of a shot of some antibiotic or other, as virtually all medications at the hospital were given by injection. The hospital did not have four hundred needles a day, however; in fact it had only a dozen or so, and the nuns used the same five needles over and over again, just swishing them around in a pan of warm water between patients.

This practice absolutely contravened good medical procedure and would not be tolerated in any well-run hospital or clinic anywhere in the world—except perhaps if you had four hundred patients that needed shots and only a few needles to inject them with. In such a situation, you practiced a sort of catch-as-catch-can, emergency medicine—it was like operating in a war zone—and so you bent the rules and hoped for the best. Besides, the Mission Hospital nuns had been doing this for years—the hospital had been operating since 1935—and there had never been a major problem with it.

Until 1976, that is, when a teacher at the Mission School came to the clinic with fever and other signs and symptoms that the nurses quickly sized up as malaria. One of the nuns gave him a chloroquine shot, the usual treatment, and sent him back out into the world at large. His problems subsided for a while but returned soon enough, and he was admitted to the hospital with high fever, bloody diarrhea, headache, chest pains, and nausea. Three days later, he died.

Back then, nobody had ever seen the Ebola virus or heard of the disease it caused, and the Ebola was a little river that flowed peacefully in a generally east-west direction about one hundred miles north of Yambuku. But the teacher would prove to be the world's first known case of what soon came to be called Ebola hemorrhagic fever.

He inaugurated two separate lines of transmission. One went from himself to his family and friends, eighteen of whom died. The virus had spread to them by means of direct contact: particles of the virus had been transferred by actual touching.

The other line of transmission fanned out from the needles he'd been injected with. Virus particles in his bloodstream had adhered to the needles as they were withdrawn from his veins, making the needle a hot object, a carrier of the virus. Those who handled the syringe afterward, such as the nuns and nurses, and those who were later injected by the very same needles, picked up particles of the virus and themselves became carriers, becoming infected, and setting up separate new rounds of transmission.

Four nurses at the hospital died of the virus, and literally hundreds of patients were unknowingly injected with it from the serial reuse of the contaminated needles. Those injections were invariably fatal, and nobody who acquired the virus by means of injection survived the disease.

In the arcane terminology of the medical profession, diseases acquired in hospitals were called nosocomial infections, from the Greek *nosokomeian*, for hospital. Typically these were caused by staph or pseudomonas bacteria, or by herpes or hepatitis viruses, and so on. The Ebola outbreak in Yambuku was something of a world-record case of nosocomial infection, as it wiped out not only many of the patients but also most of the hospital staff. "Closure of the Yambuku Mission Hospital was the single event of greatest importance in the eventual termination of the outbreak," said the official report of the World Health Organization, which investigated the case. "The epidemic waned when the hospital was closed for want of medical staff."

What was important about the Yambuku outbreak from a medical standpoint was that from the very beginning—before the virus had been identified, and before it had been named—medical people knew perfectly well how to control the further spread of it. The essential elements were nothing more complicated than standard antisepsis and barrier nursing—the use of gowns, gloves, goggles, and masks, putting an impermeable layer between the sick and the healthy.

The difference such procedures made became clear later in the outbreak when one of the nuns infected at Yambuku, Sister M.E., flew to Kinshasa together with another nun who acted as her nurse, Sister E.R., accompanied by a priest, all of whom were admitted into Ngaliema Hospital. There they were attended by South African physician Margaretha Isaäcson and a Zairian nurse by the name of Mayinga.

"From the moment of the arrival of the two nuns and the priest at the Ngaliema Hospital, Kinshasa, Zaire, on twenty-five September 1976, some precautionary measures were taken to prevent spread of infection," Margaretha Isaäcson said later. "Barrier nursing was introduced at the start, and cotton gowns and cotton masks were worn when attending the patient. These were later replaced by disposable gowns and masks, but as supplies were inadequate, the gowns and the disposable plastic overshoes were hung up outside the door of the patient's room for reuse. It is noteworthy that Sister E.R. did *not* wear protective clothing when attending her patient."

The first nun, Sister M.E., died on September 30. Eight days later the second nun, Sister E.R., who had not worn protective clothing, fell ill with similar symptoms. She died on October 14. In the entire Ngaliema Hospital, one of the biggest in the city of Kinshasa, only one other person would acquire the disease, nurse Mayinga.

Mayinga had been in contact with the first nun for several days prior to her death, and later investigators speculated that Mayinga picked up the virus in a momentary lapse of the barrier nursing procedures. Other than for her case, there had been no further transmission of the disease, despite the fact that during the time she exhibited symptoms, Mayinga spent several hours in a crowded emergency room at Mama Yemo Hospital in Kinshasa, where she shared a bottle of soda with a young boy and shared food off the plate of a fourteen-year-old girl.

From her experience with the disease in Kinshasa, Margaretha Isaäcson drew a number of conclusions. First, "it appears that the observation of the basic principles of aseptic technique or barrier nursing are probably effective in breaking the chain of infection," she said. Second, "airborne dissemination of the virus did not play a major role, if any, in the transmission of the disease." Third, "the Ebola virus is not highly infectious and requires very close contact, primarily with blood or secretions, for its transmission."

Twenty years later, those conclusions had not essentially changed. A virus, including the Ebola virus, was not something that magically tunneled through physical barriers. A layer of plastic or rubber was all that was necessary to contain it, and household bleach was sufficient to kill it.

All you had to do to prevent spread of the disease, therefore, was to erect a barrier around those infected. There was nothing arcane or mysterious about it, and neither high technology nor advanced medical knowledge was required. The underlying principle, in fact, went back more than a hundred years to Pasteur's germ theory of disease and to Joseph Lister's methods of antisepsis, both of which dated from the year 1865. The essential requirement was keeping lethal microbes away from healthy people.

Viruses were tiny molecular structures. They were impalpable and invisible to direct perception, but that didn't mean they circumvented the laws of physics. Viruses couldn't infect the healthy except by physically traveling to and entering their bodies.

If you erected physical barriers, disease transmission stopped; if you didn't, it didn't. It was that complicated and that simple.

The CDC had always had a stellar reputation for laboratory safety. There were horror stories galore about accidents in other labs the world over, but you never heard of anything untoward happening at the CDC. Apparently, its lab personnel really did have an unmatched track record for extreme carefulness, or else the accidents that occurred in its labs weren't really all that bad, or at least they weren't fatal.

All of which, if it were true, would indeed be quite surprising. After all, the laboratory technicians at the Centers for Disease Control regularly worked with a full range of the most lethal organisms, everything from rabies to anthrax, half of them causing diseases that nobody in his right mind ever heard of, such as oropouche, Sindbis, and o'nyong-nyong. The CDC was the laboratory of last resort: it was where other labs sent the pathogens that they themselves, for one reason or another, didn't want to work with, didn't have the proper containment facilities for, or were stumped by. When the Yale arbovirus lab decided to get rid of its Lassa samples in 1969, whom else did they send them to but CDC. Later, when the Pasteur Institute got a shipment of samples from the 1976 Ebola outbreak in Yambuku, no sooner did they receive the package than they got a call from Paul Brés of the World Health Organization.

"Don't open them!" he said. "They're highly infectious and must be studied in a maximum-security laboratory. They must be sent on immediately to CDC in Atlanta."

Those highly infectious agents, furthermore, were known to exert a rather unnerving metaphysical spell. People became paranoid in their presence, they became anxious and fumble-fingered. Their normally steady hands trembled and twitched, their fingers slipped, they stuck themselves with needles, they sliced into their own skin.

In 1970, when Jeanette Troup was doing an autopsy on yet another new Lassa victim, *her hand slipped,* the scalpel cut through her glove and sank into a finger, and three weeks later Jeanette Troup, too, was dead of Lassa fever.

Then in 1976, when the Prince Leopold Institute of Tropical Medicine in Antwerp got some samples of the unknown agent that had virtually rubbed out the entire hospital at Yambuku, the lab chief himself, Stefan Pattyn, was working with it, he became abnormally fumble-fingered, *his hand slipped,* and a bottle of the stuff dropped to the floor.

There were no ill effects. Still, the Antwerp lab people decided to get rid of the virus samples and sent some of them to the CDC and some to Porton Down, home of the Microbiology Research Establishment, at Salisbury, England.

The CDC, for its part, never had any accidents with it. Porton Down, however, did. When Geoffrey Platt, a technician in their highest-level biocontainment facility, held in his hand a hypodermic syringe loaded with it, *his hand slipped,* and he accidentally stuck the needle into his thumb. He contracted Ebola fever, but recovered.

No fatal self-injections ever took place at the Centers for Disease Control, and the fumbly-finger syndrome that seemed to operate elsewhere seemed inexplicably nullified here. This was all the more amazing since throughout most of its history the CDC's hot labs were thrown-together hand-me-downs cadged from other sectors of the public health system. Its very first hot lab, in fact, was housed in a sixteen-wheeler truck trailer—a moving van. It was parked out on the back lot as if it held a shipment of used furniture.

The idea behind it went back to the 1960s and to Kenneth Endicott, head of the National Cancer Institute, part of the National Institutes of Health in Bethesda, Maryland. Researchers thought at that time that some human cancers were caused by viruses, and in the event that any such cancer-causing viral agents were discovered, they thought it would be a good idea to have a secure lab facility where the pathogens could be studied in place, without the need for transport. The notion was to build a "mobile virus containment laboratory" that could be dispatched to some remote location so that the lab people could examine the agents without harm to themselves or anyone else.

The Cancer Institute therefore issued a contract to the Dow Chemical Company, whose Pittman-Moore Division, of Indianapolis, would acquire a truck trailer and convert it to a biological containment lab on wheels. Pittman-Moore purchased a stock Freuhauf trailer and had it delivered to a stainless steel—fabricating company in Orlando, Florida, which would do the actual installation work.

In Florida, workers installed safety cabinets, animal cages, pass boxes, sterilizers, fume hoods, a deep freeze and refrigerator, assorted storage units, sinks, incubators, centrifuge, autoclave, toilet, decon shower, even an air lock. They put in regular fluorescent lighting, emergency lighting, and a self-contained sewage-treatment system. The biological safety cabinets, in which the actual testing work was done, were of first quality, made by the Blickman Company of New York, who made the Class-3 cabinets that were used by USAMRIID at Fort Detrick. They came up to chest height and had glass fronts with glove ports in them through which researchers worked with the samples. The cabinets were protected by negative pressure, had provision for internal formaldehyde fumes, and other advanced features.

The trailer was air-conditioned, and completely temperature and humidity controlled, with a ventilation system that provided some twenty changes of air per hour. The air and water filtration and purification systems were so fine-grained that whatever came into or out of the trailer was pure as the driven snow. By the time it was finished, this "mobile virus containment laboratory" looked, from the inside, absolutely indistinguishable from the finest labs in use anywhere. It sparkled, it shined, it was clean as a whistle. Still, it was, from the outside, just an ordinary trailer truck, forty feet long, eight feet wide, and thirteen feet high. The price tag for all this was somewhere between $300,000 and $400,000.

No one could have foreseen, back in the planning stages, that when this beaming-white wheeled marvel rolled out of the Orlando fabrication plant in August of 1967 and headed north toward the National Institutes of Health in Bethesda, it would be at the very dawning of the African hemorrhagic fever era. The timing of it all would be a complete coincidence. But in fact the lab was emerging from its cocoon at the precise instant that the Marburg agent was doing the same thing in three cities across Europe.

The lab was somewhere in the Carolinas and on its way north when the driver received an emergency radio message from NIH. He wouldn't be bringing it up to Bethesda after all. He was to turn around and drive the lab to Atlanta, and he was to deliver it to the CDC.

A few days earlier, in Marburg, Germany, three employees of the Behringwerke pharmaceutical company had been hospitalized with an acute disease characterized by muscle aches, headache, nausea, vomiting, fever, and weakness. Simultaneously, six identical cases appeared among workers in the animal operating rooms of the Paul Ehrlich Institute, a research lab in Frankfurt. Then, two more cases cropped up at another research institute in Belgrade, Yugoslavia. The only element common to all cases was green monkeys, also known as vervets. The monkeys were routinely imported from Africa into Europe for medical research purposes, and all of the hospitalized patients had been in contact with vervets or with blood or tissue samples taken from them.

The illness and its manifestations did not fit any known disease picture, and the causal agent was quite obscure. None of the antibiotics that the doctors gave to their patients made the least dent on the course of the illness, so it was probably not caused by bacteria. "It was soon apparent," said one of the doctors, "that the infectious agent was neither bacterial nor rickettsial in origin but that a viral etiology was probable." But it did not respond to treatments for viral diseases such as yellow fever, either, and from this the doctors concluded that they were dealing with something new. For lack of a better term, they began calling it green monkey disease.

Blood samples from the patients were then offered to disease experts around the world. To them, a new and unknown infectious disease was the equivalent of an astronomer's finding a new comet or a nuclear physicist's detection of a new subatomic particle: it was terra incognita, with all the attraction of the unexplored. Samples of the "green monkey disease" agent went off to laboratories in Germany, Austria, South Africa, England, and the United States.

The Porton Down team in England had no luck in identifying the pathogen. "No definite conclusion is yet possible about the nature of the infective agent," they reported late in 1967. "The infectious agent may be an unknown organism, and further work is now required."

Some of that work was done at the CDC. The NIH trailer was stationed in the CDC parking lot back behind Building 5, a maintenance crew hooked up the high-voltage electrical feed and the water supply and waste systems, and the place suddenly had its own hot lab. A team that included Robert Kissling, chief of the virology section, Fred Murphy, an electron microscopist, and Mary Lane Martin, the technician who some twenty-eight years later would identify the Kikwit samples as Ebola, now brought the mystery agent into the lab and ran it through a battery of tests.

A defining characteristic of a new pathogen was that when tested against the antibodies for known diseases, it always yielded negative results. This proved to be true of the green monkey disease agent, which didn't react with anything at all: not with Cocal virus, Kern Canyon virus, Hart Park, nor a whole slew of arboviruses—none of them produced any reaction.

On the other hand, the mystery pathogen was observed to kill guinea pigs fairly reliably. The animals became feverish, wouldn't eat or drink, and simply lay down in their cages waiting for death. "An occasional animal developed convulsions late in the course of the disease," said Kissling. Still, some guinea pigs that had been inoculated with the pathogen and exhibited symptoms managed to survive.

The microbe also killed cells, exactly as a virus would. Starting the second day after inoculation, healthy cells began to shrink up and recoil from each other, and eventually they died and floated away. From other tests, the researchers decided that the microbe's genetic material was RNA rather than DNA, which strongly suggested that it was a virus.

Most interesting of all was what Fred Murphy saw when he viewed the diseased and dead cells under the electron microscope.

"I was a bit agitated," he said later. "This was one of the most bizarre, unearthly images ever—long filaments, 'worms,' all at fifty thousand times magnification."

Bizarre was the operative word, one that Murphy used ever afterward in a succession of technical publications about the pathogen. He spoke of seeing "many bizarre cylindrical particles," "a variety of bizarre cylindrical and fishhook-shaped particles," and so on.

They looked like the numbers 6 or 9: a long, relatively straight tail that bent around to form a loop. The particles resembled various balloon figures with a collection of weird turns, curves, bulges, and projections.

They were larger than most viruses, but came in no one regular size. "Their length varied from 130 to more than 2,600 nanometers," said Murphy. "The remarkable length and the extreme variations in the length among particles serves to emphasize the uniqueness of this agent."

It was the first of the unholy viral trio: Marburg, Lassa, and Ebola.

The fatality rate of the Marburg virus was 27 percent, which meant that you were almost three times more likely to recover from the disease than you were to die from it. This made it slightly less lethal than the most virulent strains of smallpox, some of which had fatality rates that ranged between 30 to 40 percent, and much less lethal than HIV (the AIDS virus) and untreated rabies virus, both of which had fatality rates that approached 100 percent.

But in terms of the absolute numbers of people it killed, Marburg was among the world's *least* lethal of all viruses. In its almost thirty-year history starting from the first outbreak in 1967, it had been known to kill a total of ten people. Seven of those ten had died during the virus's first appearance in Germany, and there was not another case after that for eight years. When it broke out again in 1975, in South Africa, it killed one person, making for a grand total of eight deaths due to the Marburg virus over a period of as many years. The Marburg virus, in other words, had killed an average of one person per year, worldwide, between 1967 and 1975.

A disease that killed an average of one person per year, worldwide, wasn't a public health threat by any feasible stretch of the imagination: in a given year during that same period, an average of thirty thousand people were killed by rabies, and approximately 1 million people per year died of malaria. Nevertheless, when Marburg did break out again, the CDC sprang into action. At first it was thought to be a Lassa outbreak, which was why, when CDC chief Dave Sencer got news of it, the first person he called was CDC's very own Lassa expert, Lyle Conrad.

Conrad got the call on a Saturday morning just as he and his family were on their way out the door.

"Lyle, whatcha doin' today?" said Dave Sencer, head of the CDC.

"Well, my wife and I are taking the kids up to do some camping."

"Oh, your bags are all packed, terrific! Just tell Connie you'll be a little delayed. I need you to go to South Africa."

There was a new Lassa outbreak down there, Sencer explained. An Australian hitchhiker and his eighteen-year-old girlfriend had been traveling around Rhodesia and South Africa when the guy got bit by some insect or other, developed muscle aches, nausea, and vomiting. Six days later he died. His girlfriend, along with the nurse who'd attended the hitchhiker, were now in the hospital with the same complaints. Everybody down there was sure it was Lassa. Why don't you go down there with some of Penny Pinneo's convalescent serum and see if it works?

"Just don't bring back Lassa fever," he added.

Forty-eight hours later—this was February 1975—Lyle Conrad arrived in Johannesburg. With him was a freezer box containing a vial of Penny Pinneo's blood serum, which was as much of an antidote to Lassa fever as then existed.

But the two patients, Conrad could tell as soon as he examined them, did not have Lassa fever. They had yellow fever . . . or maybe it was hemorrhagic malaria . . . or it might just possibly be hemorrhagic hepatitis. He couldn't really figure it out, their symptoms were sort of weird.

"She had a funny-looking rash, which we hadn't seen before," Conrad said of the girl. "She was dying of acute liver disease, it seemed like, or renal disease, kidney disease."

After three days of discussions with the physicians down there, Conrad got another call from Dave Sencer. Blood samples from the hitchhiker and the other two patients had been flown to Atlanta while Conrad was flying south—they'd probably crossed in flight—and the report had now come back from the lab. Sencer put Fred Murphy on the line—the electron microscopist who'd seen the Marburg agent and called it "bizarre."

"We've got the diagnosis, Lyle," said Murphy. "It's Marburg disease. We can see the bloody virus."

"I was dumbfounded," Conrad recalled. Marburg hadn't been seen anywhere in the world for eight years. On the other hand, that was all the more reason to hunt it down, find out where it had been hiding all that time.

Viruses had characteristic "reservoirs," animal, insect, or plant host species where the viruses resided more or less harmlessly between human outbreaks. Yellow fever, for example, was caused by a virus that lived in wild monkeys, who did not themselves suffer from the disease. The virus was transmitted from monkeys to humans by a separate carrier species or "vector," which in the case of yellow fever was mosquitoes.

Neither the vector nor the reservoir of Marburg virus had ever been identified, however, despite the huge searches that had been conducted in Africa immediately after the original 1967 outbreak. Brian Henderson, a CDC virologist, was part of a team that went to Uganda, where the infected green monkeys had come from, and ranged all over the country looking for them and other possible reservoir host species. They trapped hundreds of green and redtail monkeys, plus various mice, rats, and bush babies—tiny arboreal primates—and took blood, brain, liver, spleen, and kidney samples. In addition, they tracked down seventy-nine people in Uganda who'd trapped or otherwise handled the Marburg monkeys and took blood samples from them, too.

All of it went back to Atlanta. Bob Kissling and Mary Lane Martin and others tested the stuff and came up with no definitive results. For a while it looked like green monkeys really were the reservoir of the virus, and for a while it didn't. There were false positive reactions and nonspecific reactions from antibodies and other reagents, and some of the diagnostic materials turned out to be not quite sensitive enough to distinguish the Marburg agent from other viruses. Worse still, subsequent tests sometimes failed to confirm the results of the original tests, and so on and so forth. It was really a fine mess, and in the end nothing conclusive was ever established one way or another as regards the viral reservoir.

But now it was 1975 and Lyle Conrad was in Johannesburg

and he heard opportunity knocking. This was his chance to go out to the field and track down the host species of the Marburg agent, thereby becoming internationally famous and going down forever in the annals of virology.

When opportunity knocked, Lyle Conrad was not one to say no.

There now ensued one of the great virus hunts in the history of the sport as an all-star team consisting of Conrad, plus Margaretha Isaäcson, the South African physician who would stop the chain of Ebola transmission at Ngaliema Hospital in Kinshasa just a year later, plus Eric Burnett Smith, the Rhodesian minister of health, plus four other South African public health officials, now departed for the outlands. Their object was to trace back every step taken by the Australian travelers in an attempt to find how the first case, "patient 1," had been infected.

During the first two weeks of March 1975, barely a month after the two hitchhikers had originally set out, Conrad and company took the identical trip themselves. They visited each site the Australians had stopped at, looked high and low for possible animal reservoirs or insect vectors, and trapped specimens and took samples. At the end of it all they wrote up a formal account of the trip. It was an eerie day-by-day reconstruction of events, portraying the travelers at the usual tourist spots—Victoria Falls, Kyle Dam National Park, and so on—cooking their own meals, and stopping for the night at various hotels, youth hostels, campgrounds, and private homes.

1 February. They stayed overnight in a clean, well-maintained hotel, where nothing abnormal could be detected with regard to sanitation, arthropods, and food and water. They could have had indirect exposure to aerosols from insectivorous bats and fruit bats as well as to birds that nested in the attic.

There was an aviary on the hotel grounds, with pigeons,

tortoises, and rabbits, but patient 2 [the girlfriend] reported no direct contact.

At Victoria Falls, where they spent half a day, the travelers "claimed to have seen 'monkeys' at considerable distance." Conrad's team, however, spotted just one vervet there.

At a private game farm in Kyle Dam National Park, "patient 2 petted a semi-tame civet cat that had a history of being suckled by a fox terrier bitch that had simultaneously mothered two African green vervet monkeys. The team bled all of these animals as well as all game farm personnel. No significant illness had been noted before or since in animals or humans in the area."

The high point of the trip—for the virus hunters, anyway—was at a rest stop in Wankie, about fifty miles outside of Victoria Falls. This, they thought, was the scene of the crime.

Wankie. En route to Gwaai River on 6 February, the travelers spent 4 hours in the middle of the day at the Wankie roadside, waiting for a lift. A plague epizootic had passed through this area a few months earlier. While here, patient 1 [the man who died] was painfully bitten or stung on the right flank by an unknown insect, while he was sitting in the shade, up against the roadsick bank. Unfortunately, neither he nor his companion saw the insect responsible.

The site was pictured in the formal report and looked like any byway in the American West—New Mexico or Arizona, perhaps—with scrub vegetation and a few trees running up the side of a steep incline. Conrad and his crew stopped there and took specimens, all kinds of specimens.

"We trapped animals," he recalled. "We trapped rodents in particular. We trapped flies: we bought a calf and put it out there as bait to catch the flies. I bled a hundred railway workers who were working a mile away, because they'd been out there laying track for months. I bled one hundred and fifty highway workers who'd been tarring the road. The government rounded them up for me, and I bled the lot of them."

They took samples of the soil, of the plants, and of the funnel-web spiders that were abundant in the area. They packed up all these various specimens—human, animal, insect, and plant—and sent them off to the Lab of Last Resort in Atlanta . . . where nobody ever found a thing.

"Everything was negative," Conrad said. "Every animal, every person—absolutely negative."

Such results, however, never daunted the committed virus hunter. Negative results were *normal*, they were *expected*. The virus hunter, after all, was on the trail of a hidden, ghostly, almost occult adversary, and the pursuit of such game was not supposed to be easy. It was more like a military campaign or a religious crusade. It was a mythic journey, a quest, one that partook of the legendary and the fabulous. Like the heroes depicted in ancient epics and medieval verse narratives, these modern disease trackers pursued secretive antagonists in far-away and exotic lands. They courted danger and they tempted fate. They were in search of mysterious agents, shadowy evils, ancient and almost otherworldly influences.

It was a romantic adventure in the classic sense.

So now, after having failed to spy the enemy on their first attempt, Conrad and friends did the only thing they could hon-orably do under the circumstances. They went back to South Africa and did it all over again.

In June 1975, a bit more than two months after their first expedition, this same small band of disease explorers recon-vened in Johannesburg. They traveled the hitchhikers' route a *second* time, they retraced all of the hitchhikers' steps *again*, completely, minutely, inch by inch, trekking once more through the same viral outback, until they had in their various flasks, tubes, vials, and portable freezers a fine new collection of specimens.

But when that second batch of samples got back to the lab, and when the lab crew once more performed their arcane and mystic rites and rituals . . . they never found a thing.

Marburg came and Marburg went, but where it went nobody knew, not even Lyle Conrad: "That virus disappeared into the environment."

7 Ebola Fever

By 1995, almost thirty years after the initial Marburg outbreak, the press had learned all about the romance of the hot agent. Kikwit was an international media extravaganza, a story on the order of an H-bomb explosion, a major assassination, or visitors from Mars.

The press took over the Inter-Continental Hotel in Kinshasa and converted this somewhat stale and aging ten-story high-rise into a world-class communications nexus. Overnight, a clump of personal satellite dishes sprouted on the rooftop like a malignant new species of mushroom. Those little collapsible fold-open antennas, together with the transmitting hardware and battery packs that you lugged around with you in a briefcase, were mandatory equipment in the era of backwoods journalism: they beamed you up into earth orbit and put you into instant contact with any telephone, fax machine, or Internet node, anywhere in the world.

But sat-phones were only the tip of the iceberg. Reporters came to Kinshasa bearing cell phones, beepers, tape recorders,

PowerBooks, ThinkPads, modems, fax machines, digital assistants, and fabulous Nikons outfitted with all manner of advanced components: Speedlights, Multi-Control Data Backs, battery packs, chargers, motor drives, and untold numbers of autofocus zoom lenses. Broadcast journalists were in a class by themselves: entire crews—cameramen, lightmen, soundmen, fixers—pulled up to the Intercon or the Hotel Memling in vans, got out, slid back the cargo doors, and unloaded a collection of long, black, boxy containers full of lights, reflectors, tripods, booms, meters, Minicams . . .

And they did it all again the next day, when they finally arrived in Kikwit. Then they roamed through the city interviewing the townspeople, the relatives of the sick and the dead, the doctors, nurses, orderlies, Red Cross workers, the burial teams, Tamfum Muyembe, Ali Khan, and whoever else would speak to them—which even included, sometimes, other members of the press, specifically Laurie Garrett, who spent two weeks in the city.

Garrett was the author of *The Coming Plague,* subtitled "Newly Emerging Diseases in a World Out of Balance," a monumental 750-page apocalyptic tract whose ultimate message seemed to be that if we didn't soon start to "think globally," the world could shortly look forward to a fire-and-brimstone cataclysm of death by microbe.

And there it was suddenly staring them all in the face!

Well, none of this media frenzy sat too happily with the medical people, who came here to do a job, which was to stop the spread of the disease, trace it back to its first case, and look for the animal reservoir of the virus. The journalists got to be fairly annoying, especially when they showed up in the form of a mass invasion—the mob of twenty-three who burst into town on May 14, for example. This was just two days after the four viral musketeers, Rollin, Calain, Khan, and Le Guenno, had flown in. The mob came in on the Air Kasai DC-3, swarmed into the waiting vans, stopped at the hospital, the clinic, the cemetery, then got back out again posthaste.

That became a regular pattern, repeated again and again over the next several days. It got to be rather a spectacle, and even some of the press people themselves complained about it, once they got back home from Kikwit.

"Journalists were flying in from all over the world," said Laurie Garrett after she herself got back from the area. "These hordes that would show up, just horrendous! Twenty, thirty, forty journalists at once come clamoring into town and then want to have in four hours every single visual they can get their hands on. You know, the graveyard, the dying patient, the hospital, the anxious physicians, the anxious research team—then dash back to Kikwit airport, fly back to Kinshasa, and file it by satellite to their respective news organizations.

"They're crisis journalists," she added. "They fly in with their satellite dishes and their whole teams and they need the visuals and they need them now. And if they are in the way of your efforts to control the epidemic, well, too bad."

Bernard Le Guenno had particular contempt for a bunch of photographers, masked and goggled and looking much like World War I soldiers about to march through poison gas, who'd stationed themselves in the hospital courtyard where they lurked like vultures on deathwatch.

"There were two photographers, CNN with a camera and a French guy with his camera, they were waiting for three hours under the sun because there was an empty coffin outside Pavilion 3, the Ebola ward. They were waiting for the corpse—there was a nurse, a Zairian nurse who had died during the night—and they were waiting for the corpse to emerge. Three hours under the sun to have a picture of it!"

Photographers crossed safety lines with no regard for propriety or their own health. An Italian cameraman covering a mass burial crossed the ribbon barrier that had been strung up around the site and planted himself in the dirt at the edge of the burial pit about six inches away from toppling into it himself. He wore a face mask that covered his nose and mouth but was otherwise unprotected. The medical people viewed this as unbridled arrogance; still, he got some great pictures.

Worst of all in the eyes of the medics were the photographers who came into Pavilion 3 and acted as if they owned the place. They wore no safeguards and took no special pains to maintain the cleanliness of the isolation ward once sanitary conditions had been restored by Rollin and Calain. They just walked right in and started shooting.

This began with the original mob of twenty-three, one of whom, a Reuters video camerawoman, who operated out of Abidjan, Ivory Coast, was taking shots of the interior even as Philippe Calain, who had met her two days before at Kinshasa's N'Dolo airport, was asking her, *Please do not do this.* But she continued filming, at which point the quiet and monkish Calain suddenly shoved the camera away from her face. His total concern was the safety and security of his patients, whose lives he didn't want further risked by dirt being brought in from the outside, and whose illness he didn't want treated as some circus sideshow.

"Does this disease allow outsiders to forget the basic ethics of privacy and confidentiality?" he asked much later. "Just imagine that in the closest clinic here in Atlanta there's something special happening, and because of that twenty-three or maybe more African journalists come in, don't ask permission, don't introduce themselves, they open the door of the patient, see the patient lying naked, lying in blood, in stools, and they take pictures and go back out. Would people say those journalists simply 'did their job'? Nobody would agree. They would be sued."

About a week after the incident with the camerawoman, the two met up again on the hospital grounds.

"I had official permission to be there," she said later. "And I wasn't anywhere near Pavilion 3."

Nevertheless she once more bumped into Philippe Calain, who by that time had had it up to here with aggressive journalists bearing videocams. As he lurched toward her with his arms raised, she thought to herself, *My God, he's going to kill me.* He grabbed the camera out of her hands, threw it to the ground, and tried to stomp on it. She herself fell to the ground, scraping her elbow in the process.

"I lost my temper," Calain said afterward. "I regret it."

David Heymann, the WHO representative, who saw all this, cleaned and bandaged the photographer's wound, which, mild though it was, had to be taken seriously: this was prime Ebola territory and the last place in the world to sustain an injury of any sort. The camerawoman, in the end, never suffered any ill effects.

Another time, Rollin and Calain so much wanted a victim's burial to be private that they started digging the grave themselves. It was for one of the Italian nuns who'd been taking care of the patients, and who died on a Sunday evening in May. Just before sunset they placed her body in a coffin and left for the cemetery.

The cemetery was down the street from the hospital, and a nightclub was close by. When they got there with the coffin, Rollin and Calain could hear music and voices, the sounds of people dancing. Thunderclouds were rising overhead, but Pierre Rollin, dressed in street clothes, no gown, mask, or gloves, nevertheless started digging.

He didn't get far before the rain started, heavy rain that in a matter of minutes had turned the plot of ground into mud. They brought the coffin back to the convent, and the Red Cross workers buried it privately the next day.

Later, Pierre Rollin had a run-in of his own with a member of the press, specifically, Laurie Garrett. He was on his way to the hospital in Mosango where there was a separate group of Ebola patients. He was about to get into the back seat of a car to be driven away when he saw Garrett waiting there inside.

"This is my car, I'm going to Mosango," he said.

"Oh, I'm going too," she said. "Dr. Muyembe already gave me permission."

She hadn't asked Rollin's permission, though, but he let her ride with him anyway. Later, in her *Vanity Fair* account of the outbreak, Laurie Garrett would have a paragraph about herself and Pierre Rollin in Kikwit:

"I detest reporters! I will never in my life give another interview. You are a member of the lowest, most vile profession on earth," the CDC's Dr. Pierre Rollin, on loan to the U.S. agency from France's Institut Pasteur, spit at me a few days after the press invasion, although I personally had done nothing to offend him. It was my mere existence, my notebook and ancient Canon in hand, that riled the French virologist.

The French virologist himself, much later, claimed that Garrett's bird-dogging him prevented him from doing the interviewing he'd planned to do in Mosango, that in fact he'd had to make a second trip to the area to finish his work.

He also claimed, "I never said, 'I *detest* reporters.' I said, 'I *hate* reporters . . . when they behave as you do.'

"Journalists want blood, death, and screaming people," he added.

Ebola fever, however, was not confined only to journalists: it also affected the epidemiologists themselves in no small measure, and the CDC's disease hunters were no exception. They were competing to get shipped out to Kikwit with all the fury of the most scoop-hungry foreign correspondent. In fact there was a traffic jam of Epidemic Intelligence Service officers battling to go to Zaire. And why not? Every EIS officer, as part of his or her training, had to go out on an EPI-AID, an epidemic assistance detail, and the inclination within the ranks was that the more exotic the location, the better.

The EIS's own published "Guidelines for Incoming EIS Officers" boasted that "to complete EPI-AIDs, EIS officers have traveled by dogsled in Alaska, paddleboat in Bangladesh, and packhorse in the Andes. They have ridden elephants and camels in India, a helicopter over the crater at Mount St. Helens, and a military fighter in the States to deliver botulism antitoxin when a regular jet was not immediately available. Antarctica is the only continent which has not been visited by EIS officers."

So when Ebola broke out in the Congo basin, who could resist? In the disease-tracking business it was the opportunity of a lifetime, so people sent their names in to Brian Mahy, director of the Division of Viral and Rickettsial Diseases, along with a report of their qualifications, including their fluency in French, if any, asking to be shipped out. Scott Dowell, an EIS physician and extremely competent French speaker, sent his name in; Don Noah, a veterinarian, did the same; as did Peter Kilmarx, Lori Armstrong, Joe Bresee, and others. Outside the EIS, people from all over the CDC were sending their names in: Ethleen Lloyd, from the Special Pathogens Branch; Roy Baron, from the Epidemiology Program Office; even Lyle Conrad ("Uncle Lyle"), despite being on the verge of retirement and a non-French-speaker to boot, sent his name in to Brian Mahy—all of them bent on getting shipped to Kikwit.

Even those who didn't especially want to be there in person nevertheless regarded the outbreak with something other than impersonal detachment. Anthony Sanchez, the CDC lab whiz who specialized in the Ebola virus, once worried that he'd never have another epidemic to work with, no more aboriginal samples of his favorite hot agent.

"The last outbreak had occurred in 1979 in Sudan—the Sudan subtype," he said. "There was I forget how many people . . . forty, fifty, something like that, it was pretty good-sized. Since that time nothing happened, and it looked like I

131

was going to finish my career without another Ebola outbreak. It was very difficult to make progress."

But then there was Kikwit.

"This 1995 outbreak has been very positive in terms of really bringing people out of the woodwork," he explained. "A lot of people all of a sudden have an interest in doing some work on it, and this interest is expanding the directions of research: people are looking at the receptors that might be involved in the binding of Ebola virions to cells, looking at producing human antibodies, engineered antibodies, so that we might be able to protect people who have become infected."

The fact was that Ebola had been a craze among scientists from the start. Back in the original Yambuku outbreak, Pierre Sureau, the Pasteur Institute virologist, gushed while in Kinshasa, "For the community of arbovirologists, this is one of the greatest events in contemporary epidemiology. No one of us would pass up an opportunity for passionate study. Personally, I am delighted to be in this place, and to participate in such an adventure."

And so from all over the world, and not just from the CDC, virologists, physicians, and epidemiologists poured into Kikwit. David Heymann and Mark Szczeniowski, of the World Health Organization, arrived first, on May 10. Barbara Kierstiëns and Christophe Delaude, of Médecins san Frontières, arrived a day later, and the four viral musketeers a day after that. Bob Swanepoel and his assistant Felicity Burt, both of the National Institute for Virology in Johannesburg, arrived in Kikwit on May 14. Bob Colebunders, from the Institute of Tropical Medicine in Antwerp, got there on the fifteenth, along with Guénaël Rodier, from WHO in Geneva. Three experts from the Swedish National Board of Health and Welfare and the Swedish Rescue Services Agency, Bo Niklasson, Anders Tegnell, and Håkan Eriksson, came in on the seventeenth. Pierre Nabeth, a reinforcement from Médecins sans Frontières in Belgium, arrived on the nineteenth. And so on and so forth for the next three months.

In fact, David Heymann's big problem as overall coordinator of the event was keeping scientists *away* from Kikwit.

"It was one of my major concerns that there would be too many people," he said. "I was very strict with CDC, and I made some enemies there. I told them, 'No, don't send in all these people at the start, especially if they don't speak French.' There were other international partners who were coming in, and you can't discourage them from coming in by having CDC running everything. Everybody has to have a place in this, and so we wanted to make sure that the Institute of Tropical Medicine from Belgium was there, that MSF was there, that anybody who wanted to participate could participate. So we slowed down many people from coming in at the start. Later on we opened it up."

So if the scientists themselves all wanted a piece of the action, who could blame the press for their interest?

A separate problem was where to house these vast multitudes—journalists, scientists, support personnel—once they'd all arrived with their rags and baggage. Kikwit was not a place where you made "hotel reservations."

On the other hand, there *were* some hotels in the city: the Hôtel Kwilu, the Hôtel la Galette, and the Hôtel de Kikwit. From the outside, anyway, the Hôtel Kwilu was not totally implausible: it was a two-story building with rooms featuring draw draperies, sliding glass doors, and actual balconies. There were palm trees in the front, just like in Florida. The inside, admittedly, was not an exhibit of prize housekeeping skills.

"It was just incredibly dirty," said Graham Messick, chief of a CNN news team, who stayed there. "I laid out my bedroll on the top of the bed, climbed into my mosquito netting, and made sure that no part of my body ever touched the bed itself."

You hoped you could fall asleep in the heat and humidity, which were considerable. At the Kwilu, the procedure was to pay the hotel $15 extra per night in folding green American currency—this was over and above the new $25 per night room rate, up from the old $10, which had been too high even then—so that they'd keep their diesel-powered generator running for an hour or two, which in turn would keep the room fan going.

Food was its own special problem. Reporters often brought in their own food with them: crackers, nuts, canned tuna, sardines, and suchlike. The Hôtel Kwilu had its own restaurant, however, and on occasion scientists and journalists could be found there actually mixing together and contemplating the plat du jour, which turned out to be spaghetti more often than not.

"I ate spaghetti almost every meal because that's what they served," said Michael Skoler, a reporter for NPR. "They thought they were catering to European tastes."

An outsider drank only three beverages in Kikwit: bottled water, Coke, or warm beer—the famous Primus, made in Kinshasa. ("Hell, it's better than Budweiser," said one of the CDC crew.) In fact, you even brushed your teeth with the stuff, since running water—when you had it at all—came straight and unfiltered from the river Kwilu.

Despite all these protections and precautions, diarrhea was rife among outsiders (others, including Ali Khan, were constipated for days). Normally you took Lomotil for diarrhea, but this was a bad idea in Kikwit because the pills had a reputation of cross-reacting with the antimalarial prophylaxis that nearly everyone took, a drug called mefloquine. Taking the two simultaneously was thought to cause depression in some people, whereupon they stopped taking Lomotil.

The CDC scientists had most of their basic food and lodging needs taken care of well before they arrived, the arrangements for which had been made by the office of Kikwit "commandant," Ignace Mavita, the mayor.

Mayor Mavita, of course, worked in the grandest place in all Kikwit, the so-called Hôtel de Ville. This was a large white stucco building with a fine wraparound porch, located on its

own considerable plot of land behind a semicircular dirt drive-
way. His own home was also rather palatial for Kikwit, with a
living room filled with leather furniture, rugs, and shelves full
of "Ebola dolls," which is what townspeople now began calling
these traditional straw dancing figures. Once used for ceremo-
nial purposes, they were now for sale as Ebola dolls.

The place that Mayor Mavita found for the CDC team was
"George's house," which belonged to a Portuguese fish mer-
chant by the name of Jorge Quintais. It was a reasonably clean
home, concrete and cinder block, with its own screened-in
porch, three bedrooms, a living room with black vinyl furniture,
wooden tables and chairs, plus a separate dining area. There
were not enough beds to go around, so some of the CDC people ended up sharing a berth with each other just like native
Kikwitians. George's house also had a real bathroom with an
actual shower and flush toilet, above which there was an extremely large spider hanging from a web, the constant threat
of which guaranteed that nobody tarried too long at that particular bathroom fixture. What the place didn't have was a full
day's worth of running water. You had water for about an hour
or so in the morning and then again at night for some minutes,
and at those times people collected the water in pans and
bottles. The water system also functioned as an alarm clock.

"Nobody set any alarm clocks because we left all the water
taps open," Don Noah, the CDC vet, recalled. "At six or six-
fifteen in the morning the water would come on and would make
this big rushing noise. We were all programmed so that we would
just jump out of bed at that point and into the shower.

"There were eight of us in that house and the bathroom was
not as big as this room, not even close," he said, referring to
his small CDC office. "There's a sink, a commode, and the
shower. The shower is just a nozzle coming out of the ceiling,
no curtain or anything, so the typical morning there'd be some
guy brushing his teeth, some guy going to the bathroom, sitting
there, one guy in the shower standing there naked, and five

guys standing in line waiting to get the shower. So we had no secrets from each other."

George's house came complete with a housekeeper and a cook, Timothy, who made breakfast and dinner every day.

"We ate pretty well," Don Noah said. "That was a surprise. It wasn't a typical standard American menu, but we had plenty of food. We ate a lot of bread. We ate soup every day, great soup. Peanuts. Bananas. We had meat, mystery meat. Sometimes it was obvious that it was beef, and sometimes it was obvious that it was just something else.

"Everything pretty much had some gravel in it," he added. "Three of us broke teeth off. I just got back from the dentist and got the wall of my tooth rebuilt."

The samples that were sent back to the CDC, no matter where they came from, Kikwit or Kokomo, always went into the freezers.

Freezers, the place was filled with them. They were absolutely everywhere at the CDC, all over, in every corner and every corridor, and nobody who passed through its portals could escape the sight or the sound of these motionless, white, humming boxes. Even on the lower floors of the administration building—far beneath the hallowed precincts where administrators contemplated new departmental name changes and massively redundant "reorganization" schemes—there were freezers. There was no end to them. They ranged all the way from thirty-year-old double-door Kelvinator refrigerator-freezer combinations to tall gray Forma Scientific uprights, temperature minus 40° C inside, to eight-foot-long Harris freezers storing polio viruses at minus 70° C, to the ultra-cold-storage, circular CryoMed models filled with liquid nitrogen and tuberculosis. They were omnipresent at the CDC, these freezers, and the place could not live without them.

An unwholesome variety of frozen stuff was banked away

inside them, as was indicated by the red biohazard stickers that were affixed to most of the units, and as was further hinted at by the locks on some. Most of the freezers were never actually locked, however, and even of those that were, the key was often there dangling on a ribbon so that anyone who wanted to could open the door and help themselves. Not that you'd want to: labels on the sample bottles were often on the order of "Hawaii nursing home, 15 stools, 9/95," and the like. Locked padlocks and chains did exist at the CDC, but they were wrapped around the two special liquid-nitrogen units that still held smallpox virus. The more normal freezers contained the full range of chemical and biological diagnostic reagents, antibodies, convalescent serum, human and animal tissue samples, excretions and exudations of every sort, whole frozen insects, ground monkey brains, seal kidneys, necrotic livers, mushrooms, fish, plus most of the world's known viruses, bacteria, fungi, and rickettsias.

And then there was the unknown stuff.

The surprise was that CDC scientists were sometimes completely in the dark as to the biological identity of what it was they were storing away in the deep freeze. They knew where it had come from, and they knew how many cases of illness or death it had caused, they just didn't know what it *was*. Despite all the tests, despite all the microscopes, machines, and everything else, some hot agents remained unknown and unnamed for a long time.

There was the case of the St. Elizabeth's mystery agent, for example, which went back to July 1965, when eighty-one mental patients of St. Elizabeth's Hospital, Washington, D.C.'s famed psychiatric facility, came down with pneumonia. The hospital, which held a total population of about six thousand, democratically housed both the celebrated and the nameless, and for thirteen years, from 1945 to 1958, had incarcerated the poet Ezra Pound, who nevertheless managed to write the ten *Pisan Cantos* while in residence, not to mention winning the first Bollingen Prize for poetry. St. Elizabeth's was also unusual in that until just before the outbreak a pig farm was on the grounds—a charming family of penned pigs smack in the middle of the District of Columbia.

The outbreak started toward the end of July. The doctors couldn't bring it under control, however, and on August 6, 1965, the hospital administration formally requested the CDC's help in tracking down the microbe responsible. Before the epidemic was over a month later, fourteen patients would die of the disease.

The CDC sent a bunch of its EIS officers up to St. Elizabeth's, and in standard fashion they took hundreds of blood and tissue samples from the patients and sent them all back to Atlanta. In equally standard fashion, the lab crew ran the samples through the usual tests, applying the conventional selection of antibodies and reagents to positively identify the pathogen.

The samples, however, weren't cooperating. They wouldn't react with anything under the sun, they responded to none of the diagnostic materials for known diseases, viral, rickettsial, or bacterial.

Examination of the hospital grounds, furthermore, turned up some equally puzzling facts, especially when they were considered against the epidemic curve of the outbreak. That curve showed two peaks, suggesting two separate disease-causing events. The peaks corresponded to the dates when the hospital grounds were being excavated for installation of a water sprinkler system. In other words, there was a temporal correlation between the earth-moving work and the disease outbreak.

That, apparently, was a major clue, but what did it mean? Was there some mystery microbe hidden in the soil, a microbe that could suddenly become airborne, waft in on a current of air, and end up killing fourteen people?

It didn't seem likely, but the EIS disease detectives, in their painstaking, reconstruct-the-crime fashion, now plotted out the dates of rainfall in the area, the prevailing wind direction and velocity, proximity of patients to open windows, so on and so forth, and concluded in their published report that such a microbe could not be ruled out: "The etiologic agent may have resided within the soil itself, may have been deposited in sites of excavation by rodents, birds, or other animals attracted to these areas, or may have been transmitted by other unexplained mechanisms. Heavy rain followed by hot weather may have played a critical role in the spread of this disease."

Excavation, rain, and hot weather—those, somehow, were the three factors underlying the disease transmission. The identity of that "etiologic agent," however, remained absolutely impervious to every test, and so the blood and tissue samples that harbored it were lowered into the freezers at the CDC.

There they remained, immobile and untouched, for the next eleven years.

In 1968, three years after the St. Elizabeth's incident, that same microbe reared its head again, this time in Pontiac, Michigan. The circumstances were reminiscent of its first appearance—except that this time there were no deaths and it broke out not in a hospital but, embarrassingly enough, in the offices of the county health department. By actual count, ninety-five out of one hundred health department employees came down with the illness.

Once again it was the month of July, hot as blazes, when virtually the whole staff called in sick with symptoms ranging from headache and fever to shaking chills, dry cough, and chest pains. "And an air hunger," said one of the victims. "You're taking deep breaths, trying to aerate your lungs."

The CDC was called in after a week, and so on a Friday afternoon, four young EIS epidemiologists rolled into Pontiac, set up shop, and inspected the building. It was a modern, single-story affair barely more than ten years old, and contained offices, an auditorium, a library, medical and dental clinics, plus labs, storage rooms, and a small X-ray department.

By Monday morning, every last one of the EIS officers had contracted the disease themselves. "Simply being in the health

department building," one of them said, "appeared to constitute exposure."

Blood samples were taken and sent back to Atlanta where,
as before, the pathogen resisted identification. And, also as
before, the EIS team members discovered that the ground outside the building had been torn up, after which there had been
tremendous rainstorms plus a hot spell.

"During the first three weeks of June," the official report said,
"the ground adjacent to the building was regraded and paved,
which raised clouds of dust that at times enveloped the building. Torrential rains occurred the last week of June, followed
by a dramatic rise in temperature."

Excavation, rain, hot weather. In other words, they hadn't a
clue. They left the site, recovered their health, wrote up their
report, and wondered about the mysterious ways of Mother
Nature.

The samples themselves, meanwhile, were banked away in
the deep freeze where they would remain for nine long years.
Only then were they resurrected and finally identified.

When the CDC had its fatal lab accident, it was not the work
of some baffling and unknown mystery agent. It was not an
accidental needle-stick injury or a manifestation of fumbly-
finger hot-agent paranoia. It was, rather, the consequence of
a janitorial staff member's spraying down lab glassware with a
water hose. The water sprayed out of the nozzle under high
pressure, stirring up the microbes on the glassware, lifting them
up and off the bottles and flasks, creating an airborne suspen-
sion of water particles, a mist, a cloud of tiny microbe-laden
droplets that you could hardly avoid inhaling if you were
standing anywhere close . . . and within a week of that episode
two of CDC's cleanup crew were dead of Rocky Mountain spotted fever.

Not that any of this was clear at the time, the winter of 1977, and in fact the cause of the deaths was not determined until more than a week after they occurred. But then again, Rocky Mountain spotted fever was hard to detect, there being no diagnostic tests that were specific for the disease in its early stages. And so it took a full CDC investigation—the institution performing an EPI-AID on itself, essentially—before the truth, or as much of it as could be known, was established.

The two custodial men, Robert Dubignon and George Flowers, had fallen ill within a few days of each other. The first patient, a forty-nine-year-old African-American, was admitted to the Georgia Baptist Hospital on Thursday, February 24, 1977, with a high fever and rapid pulse. He was given ampicillin and penicillin. Three days later, on Sunday, February 27, he suffered cardiac arrest but was resuscitated by the doctors. He was taken to the operating room because of gastrointestinal bleeding, and he died on the operating table.

The other patient, a forty-three-year-old black male, developed a fever on Thursday, February 24, and visited the CDC employee clinic, where he was told that he had a virus of some sort and that he ought to take sick leave.

He didn't. But on Sunday, February 27, he presented himself at the Ft. McPherson Army Hospital with high fever and profuse sweating. He was admitted to the hospital, and on his second day there he had a seizure, went into a coma, and died.

The ultimate origin of the illnesses was not immediately known in either case, but in response to questioning during admittance at Ft. McPherson hospital, the second patient denied that he had been exposed to any of the microbes at the CDC. And even the CDC physician who investigated the incident, Richard E. Dixon, didn't think—at least at first—that the deaths of the two men had anything to do with the CDC's lab facilities. "My first reaction was, they should not have had any exposure to the pathogens," he recalled.

But by the time he started investigating the case, the first patient had died and the other was in a coma from which he never recovered, meaning that Dixon was never able to talk to either one. The course of events, therefore, had to be pieced together on the basis of circumstantial evidence and eyewitness testimony, like reconstructing a crime.

On March 9, test results came back showing that both of the men had died from Rocky Mountain spotted fever. This was a rickettsial disease, caused by neither viruses nor bacteria, but by a wholly separate type of organism, *Rickettsia*, named after Howard T. Ricketts, who'd discovered them around the turn of the century. Rickettsias were intermediate in size between viruses and bacteria and lived as parasites in the intestinal tracts of insects such as fleas and ticks. Typhus, trench fever, and Q fever were other diseases caused by rickettsias.

The CDC, of course, had ample stores of rickettsias on hand, including supplies of the specific subtype, *Rickettsia rickettsii*, that caused Rocky Mountain spotted fever, an acute febrile disease with a mortality rate of about 20 percent, which put it approximately on a level with Marburg fever. In one of the CDC's labs, a technician had been working with the Rocky Mountain spotted fever agent at about the time the two men became infected.

When he investigated the occurrence, Dixon found that the contaminated glassware from this technician's lab was normally taken to a holding area before it was put in the autoclave, where it was sterilized under high-pressure steam heat. In the same area, however, there was a garden hose with a sprayer nozzle attached. The first patient had been observed opening the tops of some containers and spraying down the glassware prior to putting them in the autoclave. Such a procedure, which was not standard practice and not approved by the lab safety manual, would churn up huge amounts of *Rickettsia rickettsii*.

The second patient was known to hang around with the first, and the two of them had been seen together in the autoclave room on several occasions. The second patient made a habit of collecting the aluminum-foil covers from lab glassware—also not an approved practice—and storing them in a box in his locker. The CDC investigators located the box, which indeed was full of the aluminum covers, but in a major lapse threw them away before first testing them for the pathogen. The circumstances of the case, nevertheless, added up to inhalation of *Rickettsia rickettsii* by both men, probably from the clouds of mist produced by spraying water onto infected glassware.

"How else would they have gotten the microbe?" Dixon reasoned. "They didn't inject themselves with it. They certainly didn't eat it. It must have been through inhalation."

Inhalation, moreover, would also explain why the men died so quickly. "They would have inhaled huge numbers of the organism that way," said Dixon. "And that meant a very rapid death."

The only remaining mystery was why the illness hadn't been identified in time for anyone to stop it, but there was a satisfactory explanation for that, too. For one thing, both men were dark-skinned, and the rash that was typical of the disease wasn't easily visible on a dark background. For another, it was the wrong time of year for Rocky Mountain spotted fever, which was a summertime disease: people in the Atlanta area just didn't get tick bites in February. And finally, because the men had died so suddenly, there hadn't been enough time to figure any of this out.

The incident was a low point in the history of the CDC, where people had always worked in relative safety despite being surrounded by concentrated doses of hot agents. Indeed, the only other work-related fatality in the history of the institution didn't even occur in Atlanta but rather in Nigeria, when in 1969 an EIS officer by the name of Paul Schnitker died in the crash of a plane on approach into Lagos.

The Rocky Mountain spotted fever deaths underscored the basic truth that no matter how secure a given lab facility was in itself, safety ultimately lay in the hands of the personnel who worked there. The CDC accordingly reviewed routine procedures within and outside of its various labs and made a few needed changes. A second repercussion was that the CDC officialdom now started paying some serious attention to the matter of its Level 4 biocontainment facilities, which up until this point consisted essentially of cast-off, hand-me-down portable boxes.

By the time of the Rocky Mountain spotted fever incident, the old Freuhauf trailer was long gone: it had spent only a few months at CDC during 1967—just enough time for the Marburg work to be done—before it was towed out of the parking lot and driven up to its rightful home at the National Institutes of Health in Bethesda. For a while, therefore, the CDC was left without its own separate Level 4 laboratory building. Level 4 work still went on, only it was relegated to makeshift areas inside other labs. In 1976, however, the inconceivable happened and the CDC acquired a *second* hand-me-down portable lab from NIH.

Improbable as it was, NIH now had on its hands another portable lab, a so-called "prefabricated virus concentration laboratory," which it no longer had any use for. Like its moving-van predecessor, this was another in their series of experimental movable lab facilities, one that could be built quickly at a manufacturing plant, then knocked down and carted away to be set up again elsewhere in case of emergency.

During the 1970s, the National Cancer Institute built a prototype of such a unit in the back bay of Building 41 on the NIH campus in Maryland. This new-wave transportable lab was more elaborate and less mobile than the truck trailer, but was otherwise essentially the same in plan and purpose. After setting it up in Bethesda, testing it out, and proving the general validity of the concept, the NCI was finished with the unit. It was then dismantled and sent to the CDC in Atlanta, where it was positioned on a concrete foundation in the parking lot.

The direction of travel of these throwaway labs illustrated something of the relationship between NIH and the CDC. The NIH, whose roots went back into the late 1800s and which was formally established under the name National Institute of Health in 1930, was considered to be the nation's premier public health institution. Before the CDC was ever envisioned, the NIH was already doing fundamental medical research, inquiries into the causes of cancer, and so on. The Institute had not been meant as a crisis-intervention unit, but it performed that function when necessary, sending personnel out into the field to investigate epidemics.

The CDC, by contrast, had gone out into the field from the start: its first assignment was eradicating malaria, a task that pretty much communicated the tenor and basic purpose of the place. Its primary mission was not basic research but rather controlling diseases, whenever and wherever they occurred. The two objectives were obviously related, but still there was an important distinction between them. The difference between NIH and CDC was the difference between theoretical and applied science, between abstract, "clean-hands" research versus practical, in-the-trenches, "dirty-hands" disease control.

That essential division of labor had effectively staved off any major turf battles between the two institutions. It also allowed the NIH and its associated subbranches to offer its antiquated, worn, or unneeded equipment to its somewhat dim-witted weak sister down South—or so it seemed to some of the CDC staffers who'd been on the receiving end.

Anyway, the NCI's "prefabricated virus concentration laboratory" now became the private domain of Karl Johnson, chief of the CDC's Special Pathogens Branch and the head of its Level 4 maximum-containment lab. Johnson regarded the prefabricated unit as the "thing."

"The 'thing' arrived in Atlanta in summer of '76," he remembered. "It took nearly two years for it to be outfitted and made ready for use."

Johnson was always hyperaware of the maxim that any lab was only as secure as the people who worked in it, that there was no substitute for safety awareness and correct technique on the investigator's part. His own small staff, therefore, did all of its own cleanup work and brooked no outside interference into any aspect of its operations.

"During the six years when I was at CDC," he said, "we never had a needle stick, animal bite, or major spill that caused tension in the troops while waiting out an incubation period. All staff had at least a four-year college degree, and we had no janitors or animal caretakers. The use of positive-pressure suits with individual-sized gloves to actually fit the worker, rather than cabinet lines with fixed, heavy, one-size-can't-fit-all gloves, was important in reducing the odds for invasive accidents. Aerosol control was done at the source, with good biological safety cabinets and HEPA-filtered large hoods enclosing all infected animals. The ultracentrifuge was encased in a sealed, negative-pressure filtered cabinet to prevent shrapnel and monster aerosol contamination in case of a rotor explosion.

"The point is that Level 4 can be made quite safe if thought is applied to the issues," he added, "not just a rote following of some published guideline."

Nobody ever suffered any laboratory-associated infections in either of CDC's two hand-me-down Level 4 labs. Still, it was always somewhat incongruous that an institute whose major function and reason for being was disease control would spend $12 million on a new auditorium but would consign its highest-precision, most dangerous and demanding laboratory work to modified trailers and prefabricated parking-lot marvels.

The CDC, apparently, was not averse to spending money, just to spending too very much of it on labs. Starting with the 1977 Rocky Mountain spotted fever incident, however, that attitude would change.

8 Patient Zero

According to the earliest reports reaching the outside world in May of 1995, the first human victim of the Kikwit outbreak—the index case—was a man by the name of Kimfumu.

Kimfumu was a thirty-six-year-old laboratory technician who lived in a thatched hut at Kamutsha 13 in the Nzinda zone of the city. He lived there with a sister by the name of Abimia. He'd worked at Kikwit's other hospital, Kikwit 2, also known as Mama Mobutu Maternity Hospital, a low-slung, whitewashed, tin-roofed building located a couple of miles west of Kikwit General. It was a smaller hospital than Kikwit General, with about seventy beds. At Kikwit 2, Kimfumu worked in a lab in one corner of the building, a small room with white walls, a concrete floor, and white gauze curtains covering the windows.

The lab was rather poorly equipped, with no equipment to speak of other than for a small alcohol burner that produced a flame for sterilizing instruments or heating reagents in test tubes. Over against the wall were shelves bearing an assortment of bottles containing the reagents, and next to the shelves there was a white porcelain sink above which was a single spigot. Water rarely ran from the spigot, though, and so hospital workers collected rainwater in cisterns and brought it to the lab in plastic buckets.

Kimfumu worked in the lab with another technician by the name of Bienge. A long, white lab bench ran along one wall, with two wooden stools in front of it, and Kimfumu and Bienge would sit there at the bench and run tests on the blood samples taken from the hospital patients. They did not always wear gloves when working with the samples, many of which had come from suspected shigella cases, and on April 6, Kimfumu fell ill with a fever. Two days later he was admitted to the hospital in which he worked. At first the doctors thought he had typhoid fever, but his condition soon worsened to include a distended stomach, which they took for a sign of a perforated intestine, a condition that required an immediate operation. At that point Kimfumu was transferred to Kikwit General, where there were operating rooms and appropriate surgical staff.

The operating rooms at Kikwit General were in Pavilion 7, which was just behind the emergency room and diagonally across the grassy center courtyard from Pavilion 3. Pavilion 7 was normally closed to outsiders, and the entrance to it was barred by a locked red metal gate. Kimfumu would be operated on in Salle B, a small blue cubicle with a gray ceramic-tile floor. Standing approximately in the center of the room in front of two glazed windows was a flat metal surgical table set on a hydraulic lift whose height was controlled by means of a foot pedal, like a barber's chair. The patient's position was further adjustable by means of a hand crank located at knee level. On top of the metal platform, which showed some rust, lay a thin red plastic mattress and a slightly thicker red plastic pillow. Around the table were racks that held surgical instruments, sterilization equipment, and supplies. A large white operating lamp hung from the ceiling.

On Monday, April 10, 1995, Kimfumu was wheeled into Salle B, induced into unconsciousness by the anesthetist, and operated on by a team of two doctors assisted by two nurses. They performed a laparotomy, a standard procedure for opening the abdomen, and found that Kimfumu was suffering from an inflamed appendix, which they removed. For a while he seemed to be recuperating, but the next day his midriff was even more bloated than before, and a second surgical team performed a repeat laparotomy. This time the abdominal cavity was filled with blood, and the internal organs were disgorging themselves of vital fluids and bleeding out into his open belly. Kimfumu's blood went all over the place and spattered the gowns of the doctors and nurses. The patient subsequently went into shock, and on April 14 he died.

Then, one by one, so did several members of the operating teams. Sister Floralba, one of the nurses, fell ill with fever, headache, and external bleeding and was transferred to a larger and better hospital at Mosango, some eighty miles away. She died there on April 25. Jean Kingansi, a male operating-room nurse, and Willy Mubiala, an anesthetist, soon presented the same clinical symptoms, were hospitalized, and both of them died in Kikwit on the twenty-sixth. Additional cases spread out from there along a line of transmission—which Ali Khan soon began referring to as a "chain of death"—that had sprung from Kimfumu, who now appeared to have been a viral time bomb who had exploded with Ebola particles and scattered them all over the hospital.

That was an accurate enough picture as far as it went, but in fact the chain of death in Kikwit had started long before Kimfumu had taken sick. Bienge, Kimfumu's thirty-year-old co-worker in the Kikwit 2 lab, had entered the hospital on April 7, a day before Kimfumu, with fever, headaches, bloody diarrhea, abdominal distension, asthenia, and "red eye." Both of them died on the same day, April 14.

But there had been even earlier cases, as Tamfum Muyembe

learned when he came to Kikwit to investigate the epidemic. For three days he pored over hospital records and pieced together the chronology of events, and on May 4 he wrote up a brief account of his findings:

> In the reference case, Bienge was infected by the same source as Kimfumu, both laboratory assistants at KK2. Bienge died at KK2 while Kimfumu died at the General Hospital on the same day (April 14, 1995). Both laboratory assistants might have been infected by blood (while taking it or while handling it in the laboratory) from patients who came for a medical examination at Kikwit 2. This was the case of:
>
> 1. Kawenga, head of personnel of KK2, deceased on April 12, 1995.
> 2. Kimbambu, transferred to HGK [Kikwit General Hospital] and deceased on March 27, 1995.
> 3. Kifoto, caretaker of Kimbambu, deceased on April 4, 1995, at HGK.

But they, too, were only the tip of the iceberg. Well before Muyembe arrived in Kikwit, Dr. Kiyungu-Kambidi, the medical director of Kikwit 2, had noticed a sharp rise in the number of deaths at his hospital. In the month of January there had been no deaths at all, in February there was one, in March, three, and then in the first three weeks of April alone, six patients had died. Dr. Kiyungu-Kambidi had himself tracked the progress of these cases with exceptional care, and before the month of April was out he had produced a fifteen-page typewritten report documenting the evolution of the cases, listing the drugs and other treatment the patients had received, and giving their final outcomes.

Then, entirely on his own, Kiyungu-Kambidi concluded that an outbreak of some sort was in progress, one that he identified as "an apparent epidemic of hemorrhagic gastroenteritis," a condition that he said "leads rapidly toward death." Then he formulated a comprehensive plan to deal with the situation, one that included informing the city's population of the danger, encouraging them to adopt strict sanitary procedures at home—washing their hands before eating or drinking, boiling water before use, and so on—and advising them to bring all suspected cases of the disease to the hospital. The plan, had it been put into effect, would probably have reduced the severity of the epidemic even if it might not have stopped it.

Finally, on April 24, two weeks before the Kikwit blood samples had left Brussels for Atlanta, medical director Kiyungu-Kambidi photocopied his fifteen-page report and sent it out, along with a cover letter, to various relevant parties including the minister of public health in Kinshasa, the regional medical inspector of Bandundu province, Mayor Mavita in Kikwit, the director of Kikwit General Hospital, the local Kikwit representatives of Oxfam, the World Health Organization, and UNICEF. He even sent a copy to the head of the local Lions Club.

And then, at that critical juncture in the development of the Kikwit outbreak, when a forceful intervention could have made a massive difference to the end result . . . nothing happened. If anyone read his report, apparently nobody paid the least attention to it. In any event, no one seemed to have followed it up. "This report was sent to everybody but received by nobody," said Bernard Le Guenno.

Kikwit General Hospital now became the focal point and main amplification center of the Ebola virus. The hospital was like the hub of a wheel with spokes radiating out from the core: patients would be brought in through one of the spokes, they'd erupt with the virus, infecting family members and hospital staff alike, and then these infected people would exit the hub through other spokes, where they would in turn infect others. Later they'd reenter the hospital as patients themselves, they'd explode in a fresh new rain of virus particles, and the cycle would start all over again. The hospital, meanwhile, periodically relieved itself of its dead by pouring the corpses out into a hole in the ground, a mass grave.

That was how the place operated, anyway, until just before the arrival of the CDC. By that point, both the hospital staff and ordinary townspeople had taken the place for a death house. They regarded it as an exit door from earthly life, a building from which anyone who entered was not likely to walk out again. That was why the hospital was deserted when the CDC's first foot soldiers got there and walked through the grounds: the medical staff had disappeared and family members no longer visited the patients.

But the place seemed to function in that same way even after Pierre Rollin and Philippe Calain got there, cleaned it up, instituted sanitary measures and barrier nursing procedures, and put an end to hospital-based virus transmission. The hospital remained a death cell, the reason being the lag time between the stoppage of transmission and the point where the effect showed up in the form of lower mortality rates. And the reason for this, in turn, had to do with the incubation period of the virus, which ranged anywhere from two days to three weeks. You could put an end to new transmission on day one and still have new cases showing up two to three weeks later.

It was no particular surprise, then, that the city's highest death toll corresponded to the CDC's arrival in Kikwit. On May 12, the very day that Calain, Rollin, Khan, and Le Guenno landed at Kikwit airport, there were fourteen new Ebola deaths. Almost two weeks later, on the twenty-fourth, there were ten new deaths, which contributed to the impression that the epidemic was rolling along of its own accord despite everything that the medics had done to stop it. When sixty people died in a single week, even the normally self-possessed Ali Khan suffered a rare crisis of confidence. "I really began to worry about the whole thing getting out of control," he said.

It was his unenviable task to persuade new cases to admit themselves voluntarily into the hospital. This had to be done because it was the only way, short of evacuating the whole city, of isolating the sick from the healthy. But coaxing the victims into Kikwit General was no easy matter.

"There was all sorts of resistance, people who didn't want to go to the hospital," Ali Khan said. "There was a guy who was found hiding in a barrel at his second wife's house, people hiding other cases. For a lot of people, the outbreak was associated with the hospital, and the hospital was where you went to die."

And who could blame them? The families who brought their loved ones to the hospital usually saw them emerge a few days later wrapped in a white body bag. They'd stand there and watch from the grassy courtyard as two or three Red Cross workers, spooky figures in greenish blue smocks, white aprons, helmets, and gloves, wheeled a gurney bearing their father, mother, sibling, or child out of the isolation pavilion, down a covered walkway, then out onto a dirt path leading toward the morgue building.

Later, a yellow Renault dump truck would slowly back up to the morgue and six or seven of those same blue-suited figures would jump down from the truck, enter the morgue, pull the bagged and nameless bodies out of the darkness, and heave them up onto the truck bed. There they'd lay, lurching back and forth with the truck's motions as it drove toward the cemetery.

Where, finally, you saw your father or mother, sister or brother, lowered into the burial pit. They'd be dropped into the pit along with the others, and then a bulldozer, another massive yellow piece of equipment, would fire up, steam forward, and push a pile of mounded-up dirt back over the bodies.

That's what happened to your loved ones when you brought them into Kikwit General. Some two hundred people would go into the hospital alive and come out in body bags in just that manner, which was why people fled to other cities or hid in their homes or sometimes tried to treat themselves. One Kikwit pharmacist set up an intravenous drip for himself at home: he tacked the IV bottle to the wall above his bed, stuck the needle into his arm, and watched and waited. He was found dead on a thin, blue mattress on the concrete floor, a red bloodstain surrounding his head like a halo.

A former Zairian Army sergeant died in his home and was buried in a shallow grave in his backyard. Another victim, it was said, died in his outhouse, and his body slumped down into the opening and fell to the bottom. It was left there and buried just as it landed.

And some victims, despite everything, actually allowed themselves to be brought to the hospital. Since there were no ambulances, they came from their homes by any means available, sometimes in the back of pickup trucks. Others arrived from Kikwit 2, the maternity hospital, in trucks, private cars, or in taxis. One patient was put into a taxi at Kikwit 2 but died before reaching Kikwit General. When the hospital attendants opened the taxi door, the corpse fell out onto the grass.

Events had taken a different course the first time Ebola hemorrhagic fever had appeared in the developed West. It had happened in London in 1976, shortly after the original outbreak in Yambuku.

It was the case in which Geoffrey Platt, a lab researcher at Porton Down, the British biological research center, was working with Ebola samples that had come in from Yambuku. He was injecting a guinea pig with a syringe loaded with the virus when all of a sudden *his hand slipped* and the needle went into his thumb. Within a week he had the fever himself, the first human case of Ebola disease ever to appear in Europe.

Geoffrey Platt was thereafter treated as if he were a piece of nuclear weaponry or an alien visitor from outer space. He was given a respirator mask to breathe into so as to keep the virus away from others. He was put into an ambulance, surrounded by a cordon of bobbies on motorcycles, and taken by caravan to the infectious diseases unit at Coppetts Wood Hospital in North London.

In Coppetts Wood, at the time, 160 other patients were snug in their beds. All of them were removed from the hospital and taken to other institutions elsewhere.

In a building now empty of patients, Geoffrey Platt was placed into a room in the highest-security area, then further enclosed inside an additional protective barrier membrane, a Trexler negative-pressure plastic isolator. This was a tent of transparent film whose internal pressure was kept below that of the surroundings so that contaminated air would be prevented from bleeding out of it. Air was drawn into the canopy from the outside, then drawn out again by fans, then passed through a series of HEPA filters—high-efficiency particle arresters—before finally being exhausted out of the building above roof level. Alone inside his quarantine capsule, Platt was so completely sealed off from the rest of the world that he might as well have been on planet Jupiter.

Food, medications, and other supplies were passed into the canopy through an entry port without breaking the pressure seal. Infected material was put into sealed plastic bags and conveyed out of the tent in the same way. Dry waste was incinerated; liquid waste was chemically disinfected, then boiled, and then released into the sewer system.

He was kept in his tent for thirty-two days, tended round the clock by a medical staff consisting of five doctors and twenty-four nurses, all of whom, despite the fact that they were physically separated from the patient by the plastic isolator and negative air pressure, were themselves placed under quarantine for the duration.

Porton Down, meanwhile, was shut down and the staff was sent home, and for a time the place was regarded as an infectious death trap glowing with some mysterious and unknown viral radiation. Simultaneously, the more than three hundred people with whom the patient might have been in contact prior to being isolated were hunted down by public health officials, questioned, and placed under surveillance for possible signs of Ebola fever.

And then, finally, Geoffrey Platt recovered. He left the isolator and was placed into another high-security room in the same hospital. The room he'd been in was now invaded by staff members dressed in space suits and biological respirator units. The spacemen put a couple of electric heaters on the floor, set open containers of formaldehyde on the heaters, and left the room. Twenty-four hours later they reentered the sealed room, aired it out, and dismantled the isolator canopy. They removed it, fumigated the room a second time, and sealed it back up again.

Then they set the canopy ablaze.

"The canopy was in fact too large to go through the opening of any of the incinerators we had," said one of the doctors. "So rather primitively, we dug a hole in the field and burned it."

And after that, Coppetts Wood Hospital, Porton Down, and Geoffrey Platt himself, all slowly returned to normal.

About a year later, in December 1977, the Prince Leopold Institute of Tropical Medicine in Antwerp sponsored a conference on Ebola fever. The doctor who'd been in charge of Geoffrey Platt's case in London, Ronald Emond, gave a presentation describing the course of treatment, use of the plastic isolator, the quarantine of staff members, and so on. In the audience were several of the medical people who'd participated in the 1976 Yambuku epidemic, including Margaretha Isaäcson, the South African physician who'd treated Nurse Mayinga at Ngaliema Hospital in Kinshasa, and the CDC's own Karl M. Johnson, chief of the Special Pathogens Branch, who'd been at Yambuku. Even after having been in the middle of the outbreak themselves, however, both of them were somewhat taken aback by the strictness of the measures applied in Platt's case.

"What would be wrong with disinfecting the isolator with ethylene oxide and reusing the canopy?" asked Margaretha Isaäcson.

"The total cost for this particular episode was so enormous," said Ronald Emond, "that the canopy was negligible in it. If you consider that all the scientific staff in Porton were put off work and under surveillance, that our hospital with one hundred and sixty people was put out of action, and that a great many community physicians were involved, the total cost must have run into one hundred thousand or two hundred thousand pounds. The price of the envelope is about nine hundred pounds sterling."

Karl Johnson asked, "Why was it deemed necessary, even in the beginning, to quarantine medical staff that was protected by the bed isolator?"

"In Great Britain, as in other countries," said Emond, "there was considerable panic at the reports that were coming from Africa about this new disease. The equipment at that time, although it had been used on a considerable number of occasions, had never been used in any really serious infection. Thirdly, one of the patient's children developed a mild fever and it was thought possible that it was going to spread within the family grouping. Taking all things into consideration, it was thought advisable that the staff should be asked to go into voluntary quarantine, which they agreed to do."

Considerable panic, evidently, could be expected to accompany any case of Ebola fever that ever reached the civilized West. But if Geoffrey Platt's treatment was any indication, that panic was largely misplaced. Lurid horror stories to the contrary, Ebola was not a disease that was going to rip through the Western world unchecked while its medical forces and public health networks stood by and watched, mute and helpless.

Patient Zero of the Kikwit outbreak was not Kimfumu or Bienge or anyone else who'd been in Kikwit 2 maternity hospital, whether as caregiver or patient. Patient Zero was a thirty-five-year-old charcoal maker and manioc farmer by the name of Gaspard Menga.

Ali Khan had heard rumors about him time and again during his traceback work. Khan himself focused on the epidemiology of the outbreak, tracing back the lines of transmission that would lead to the genuine index case, one that could not be followed back any further and prior to whom there were no suspicious deaths. In this he had the help of students from Bandundu University, a medical college in the city not far from Kikwit General. They'd meet in the morning at the headquarters building, get their assignment, pick up a sheaf of standardized questionnaires, then disperse out into the city on a variety of motorcycles, scooters, bikes, cars, pickup trucks, and on foot, to locate and question surviving family members. It was plain and classic shoe-leather epidemiology.

"It's the routine stuff we do that we're taught at CDC," said Ali Khan. "It's not very glamorous in any way, shape, or form, but it's critical and vital to everything that happened."

Not long after starting the traceback, they'd heard stories about a family who, months earlier—maybe March, maybe February, maybe even as far back as January—had been just about completely wiped out. A dozen or so family members had died, one after another, for no known reason, just like that.

The family had lived in Kikwit in a pretty area in a large and long yellow building set back against a small hill. A cluster of tall palm trees overhung the house. Before Gaspard Menga took sick, more than twenty family members had lived there.

Menga was a tall, serious-looking man who wore a mustache and neatly trimmed beard. He'd been baptized a Seventh-Day Adventist only a couple of years earlier. He made a living by cultivating a manioc plot and making charcoal in the Pont Mwembe forest, about eight or ten miles from Kikwit. It was an extremely hard occupation as it required his making long daily bike rides over a bad and rutted dirt road that wound its way into the jungle. To make a single load of charcoal took some three months from start to finish, for a payment that came to about three dollars' worth of zaires, the national currency.

On January 6, during the height of the rainy season, Gaspard Menga developed a fever, bloody diarrhea, and abdominal pain. He was admitted to Kikwit General Hospital, where he was diagnosed as having shigella, the bacterial disease whose symptoms somewhat resembled the early signs of Ebola fever. But a week later, on January 13, he died.

There was an open-casket funeral, which was traditional in the area, and a principal vehicle by which the virus would spread through the city before the medical team members put an end to the practice. In Menga's case, family members had crowded around the open casket and placed their hands on Gaspard Menga one last time, in sign of affection and farewell. His wife, Bebe, his brother, Bilolo, his uncle, Philemond—all of them touched the body of Gaspard Menga as it lay there in the open casket . . . and all of them died shortly thereafter. On January 29, Philemond died at Kikwit General Hospital. Two days later, so did Gaspard's brother, Bilolo, and on that very same day, Gaspard's wife, Bebe, died at home.

That was the first wave of death: Gaspard and the three who'd touched his dead body. But then there was a second wave, which consisted of sisters, sons, daughter, and grandmother, all of whom died in February. Then there was a third wave, the last of whom, a grandmother, died at home on March 3, in the outlying village of Ndobo.

And there, for no immediately apparent reason, the chain of infection terminated. It simply stopped, it halted abruptly of its own accord, in circumstances that were otherwise highly favorable to continued transmission: those who'd died had been in close proximity to many others who yet lived on in perfect health. As had been true in the earlier Ebola outbreaks, chains of transmission ended on their own, without benefit of medical intervention or anything else.

A separate line of transmission, however, found its way into Kikwit 2 maternity hospital, where a friend of the Menga family was admitted, and who died there on March 3. The victim was one of the three deaths to have occurred in that hospital in the month of March.

In the end, Ali Khan, Bernard Le Guenno, and their small army of helpers would be able to trace the whole Kikwit outbreak forward from Gaspard Menga. They'd construct a complex diagram of the outbreak, with arrows pointing from the Mengas to new cases, from whom other arrows pointed to an ever greater number of victims.

But they could not trace it back an inch further. The unanswered question, then, was: Where had Menga gotten infected? And from what person, animal, insect, or plant?

Never once in the history of either disease had a hunt for the reservoir of Marburg or Ebola been successful. When Lyle Conrad and his friends from South Africa had made their two consecutive trips through the outback looking for whatever it was that had transmitted Marburg virus to the Australian hitchhiker, they'd failed to find a hint of it anywhere. After several weeks of searching, trapping, drawing blood samples and sending them to Atlanta, their formal and final conclusion was: "The reservoir and possible vectors of the disease remain unknown."

The situation had not changed in the least twenty years later despite two fleeting appearances of the Marburg virus, both of them in Kenya, in 1980 and 1987. Only one person died in each instance, but in the spring of 1988 researchers from USA-MRIID, the U.S. Army's infectious diseases unit at Fort Detrick, Maryland, nevertheless launched a major international expedition to Africa, to what they thought was the probable home of the mystery virus: Kitum Cave on the side of Mount Elgon in western Kenya. They went out there and in space suits and respirators trapped flying insects, ticks, mice, birds, bats, rats, cats, and a few other miscellaneous animals—everything, it seemed, but the fabled virus itself, of which they found absolutely no trace whatsoever.

Following that wild-goose chase, there had been no reports of new Marburg cases anywhere in the world, which meant that by mid-1996 it still remained true there had been only ten known deaths in the disease's thirty-year history. This made it one of the rarest infectious diseases of all time. Indeed, more people had walked on the moon than were known to have died of the Marburg virus.

Ebola was more lethal than Marburg both in terms of its mortality rate as well as the total number of deaths it caused. Still, from the time of the first Ebola epidemics in 1976 through the beginning of 1996, a period of almost twenty years, there had been fewer than 700 known deaths due to the virus, for an average of 35 deaths per year, worldwide. When measured against a global population of some 5 billion people, that was not an especially huge number. How small a number it actually was could be judged by comparing it against figures for almost *any* other agent of death. The CDC's own National Center for Health Statistics recorded that during the time the Ebola virus was killing some 700 people worldwide, a total of 2,698 people in the United States alone—more than 100 people per year—had been killed by "lightning, lightning shock, stroke, or thunderbolt." (Nobody spoke of lightning as "the revenge of the thunderclouds," even though there was abundant talk of Ebola as "the revenge of the rain forest.") The CDC's records showed, in fact, that while an average of 35 people per year were killed by Ebola across the globe, an average of 300 people in a single country, the United States, died each year by "drowning, submersion in bathtub." In 1991, 1,247 people in the United States died of "inhalation or ingestion of food," meaning that in a single year in one country, more people choked to death on food in their own homes than were known to have died from the Ebola virus in all of history.

As for the Ebola virus itself, it was so extremely rare and elusive a microbe that when groups of trained researchers set out to locate examples of it in its known haunts—which was to say, in the rain forests—they failed utterly in every attempt, time after time. Unequivocally, it was far easier to find diamonds in Africa than it was to find the Ebola virus. Marburg and Ebola, therefore, were rarities in the extreme; they were more in the nature of medical curiosities than they were significant threats to public health.

Lassa fever, on the other hand, the third member of the unholy trio, presented quite a different picture. It was far and away the most lethal of the unholy trio in terms of the absolute number of deaths it caused: "Three thousand to five thousand Lassa fever deaths occur each year in West Africa," said the CDC's Karl M. Johnson. That *was* a significant public health threat, and finding the reservoir or vector of Lassa fever was a matter of some urgency. It would let you advise people to take measures against the guilty animal or insect, and thereby reduce the number of additional cases. And so in 1972, when a new Lassa epidemic broke out in Liberia, the CDC sent Tom Monath, a Harvard M.D. and virologist, to Zorzor, site of the outbreak, to trace back through the chain of transmission for the index case and also to search for the host organism of the Lassa virus.

Zorzor turned out to be another hospital-epidemic horror story. The outbreak started when a young Liberian woman came to a clinic with a cluster of hemorrhagic fever complaints: fever, vomiting, abdominal pain, and bleeding. Shortly after being admitted to the hospital, she suffered a miscarriage of the twin fetuses she'd been pregnant with, after which a missionary nurse performed a dilation and curettage, a routine procedure she'd done many times before.

The woman recovered and returned home to the town of Zigida. At the hospital, meanwhile, eleven other patients fell ill with the same clinical signs and symptoms, and five of them—including two nurses—had died.

Tom Monath now arrived in Zigida, tracked down the woman, and took blood samples from her as well as a hundred other villagers. She and four others turned out to have Lassa antibodies, meaning that all of them had been infected by the virus, so Monath hired a bunch of hunters from the village and went out with them at night to set traps for mice, rats, and bats—the three most likely suspects. In the mornings they'd find an average of twenty trapped animals, and then, outfitted in gloves, gown, and mask, they'd anesthetize and sacrifice them, cut them open and extract blood and various sections from internal organs, all of which was put into Vacu-tainer tubes and placed on ice.

They did this for eight days in a row, coming back with samples from 164 separate animals. Then Monath sent the specimens, bottled, bagged, and tagged, to Atlanta . . . where it was of course discovered, as was absolutely predictable, that not a single one of them contained any trace of Lassa virus.

After a second outbreak a few months later in Sierra Leone, Monath and some others from the CDC—David Fraser, Paul Goff, and Kent Campbell—went over there and did it all over again. This time they trapped four times as many animals as before, for a grand total of 641, including eight rats that they'd taken from the house of a patient who'd died. The house was overrun with ten-inch-long, brownish gray rodents, members of the species *Mastomys natalensis*.

It wasn't until some nine months later, in June of 1973, that Monath, back at the CDC, finally got around to testing them. The specimens had been in the deep freeze the whole time, and he'd been testing the other stuff first, but when he finally defrosted the *Mastomys* sections, ground them up with mortar and pestle, and spread them out across the culture medium, lo and behold they proved to be saturated with Lassa. It was a historic moment, a milestone at the CDC, and it represented a major advance in the epidemiology of the disease.

The only thing it didn't do, unfortunately, was have any effect on the frequency of new outbreaks, which continued on pretty much as before. Discovering the reservoir of a given virus did absolutely nothing to stop further outbreaks of the disease it caused, nor did it make those outbreaks less severe, nor did it save the lives of those affected. Abstract knowledge had to be accompanied by practical action, and practical action was not always forthcoming from the governments or public health authorities of the nations at risk, or from the people themselves, for that matter—as the later history of Lassa would quite clearly illustrate.

Sixteen years after its rodent reservoir was identified, and twenty years after Lyle Conrad first brought the disease into the country, Lassa fever paid a repeat visit to the United States.

It was February 1989, height of flu season, and half the population of Glen Ellyn, Illinois, a Chicago suburb, seemed to have caught the bug. So when a forty-three-year-old black mechanical engineer showed up at an urgent care center with a temperature of 101° F, chills, sore throat, and muscle aches, what else could it be but the flu? As they told you in med school, "If you hear hoofbeats in Central Park, don't expect zebras."

The man was given a prescription and was sent home. His condition failed to improve, however, and about two weeks later he was admitted to Central DuPage Hospital in Winfield, Illinois, where he was placed under "universal isolation precautions," which essentially meant barrier nursing. The precautions had been developed by the CDC in 1987 as a way of preventing hospital transmission of blood-borne diseases such as AIDS and hepatitis B, and they amounted to the use of gloves, mask, and goggles when dealing with a patient's blood or bodily secretions. The patient had been put under these safeguards since the hospital's admitting physician had now given a tentative diagnosis of hepatitis and/or possible yellow fever.

The next day, an infectious disease specialist by the name of Bob Chase examined the man and spoke to his wife, who told him that her husband had recently come back from Nigeria where he'd gone to attend his mother's funeral. His mother had supposedly died of malaria—or at least that was what the Nigerian doctors claimed. But during his stay in the country, several of his other family members had also come down with illnesses, including the patient's father, who also died.

None of what Bob Chase heard from the wife, nor what he saw in the patient in front of him, who was oozing and bleeding and had bloody diarrhea, added up to malaria. It sounded like an African hemorrhagic fever, and so he placed a call to the CDC in Atlanta.

He talked to none other than Joe McCormick, the mythic chief of the Special Pathogens Branch and the successor to Karl Johnson. McCormick listened to the patient's history and signs and symptoms and promptly told Chase that he was dealing with Lassa fever. McCormick also told Chase he'd be there the next day, and that in the meantime he'd try to get the CDC's portable isolation unit flown to Chicago. Approximately three hours after that telephone conversation, though, Chase's patient died.

But McCormick showed up the next day as scheduled, along with Gary Holmes, an officer of the Epidemic Intelligence Service. They'd brought a bunch of reagents and antibodies along with them, and when the patient's blood and liver samples were tested against them, there was no doubt he'd died of Lassa. The question was, what to do about the dead man's wife and their six kids, who'd been in direct contact with him every day from the time he came back from Africa until he'd entered the hospital. They'd cared for him at home, eaten food from his plate, cleaned his bed linens, and so on. Plus, lots of other people had associated with the patient during those two weeks.

But Holmes and McCormick had the situation well in hand. They gave an antiviral drug, ribavirin, to the patient's family, who were at the highest risk for the disease, and then with the cooperation of state and local health workers, they set up a standard traceback and surveillance system to follow up the hundred or so persons who'd been in contact with the patient during the time he was likely to have been infectious.

No one else in Glen Ellyn contracted Lassa fever. As had been true in Geoffrey Platt's case, the epidemic had been stopped by human intervention before it ever began.

These African hemorrhagic fever viruses, apparently, were easy enough to contain so long as you were aware that you were dealing with them, and so long as you had the resources, manpower, and know-how to bring to bear on the situation. You also had to acknowledge that a Lassa outbreak was actually occurring, instead of disguising it as something else—such as malaria, for example.

"Malaria was a surrogate diagnosis," said Gary Holmes of the Illinois case. "The health officials in Nigeria just didn't want to admit there was another Lassa outbreak in the country."

The virus itself, in other words, wasn't so much the problem. Human behavior was more the problem.

9 The Forest

Apocalyptic thinking was a rare occurrence at the Centers for Disease Control, but it was not a wholly unknown activity. Isolated outbreaks of infectious diseases, after all, could and did escalate into major epidemics, and major epidemics killed millions of people, and an ounce of prevention was worth a pound of cure, especially when the diseases in question *had* no cure, which, despite all the progress that had been made against them, was still far too frequently. All of that was perfectly true. Nevertheless, matters got entirely out of hand starting on Saturday, February 14, 1976, Valentine's Day, when Dave Sencer, head of the CDC, called an emergency meeting to consider the recent bad news from New Jersey. An apparent case of swine flu had cropped up on the Fort Dix Army base, and the victim, an eighteen-year-old recruit, had died.

Influenza was bad enough when what you were dealing with was a case of ordinary, "benign" flu such as often appeared during the winter and killed an average of twenty thousand Americans in a given year. That was the seasonal death count

167

of an average flu strain: twenty thousand American dead, period.

And that was for an *ordinary* flu, garden-variety. Swine flu was exceptional because it was similar in its molecular structure to the strain that had been responsible for the influenza pandemic of 1918 in which approximately 21 million people died, including half a million Americans. In New York City alone, there had been some twenty thousand influenza deaths in 1918. According to tests done initially in New Jersey and then repeated at the CDC, the virus strain responsible for the Fort Dix case was closely related to the influenza that had gone round the world in 1918, and it had already caused one death. Few people alive in 1976, sixty years later, would have antibodies to the original virus, which meant that the stage was set for a major epidemic.

Maybe. The problem was that flu viruses were highly unpredictable; they came and went of their own logic, a calculus that was neither fully understood nor amenable to trustworthy extrapolation. The viruses mutated and changed and reassorted their molecular elements; they passed from one host species to another; they hid out in the environment; they traveled aloft in ducks and geese that sailed hither and yon in the wind; and the final upshot of all these combined movements and imponderables was not really knowable in advance of its happening.

In addition to which there was the matter of "cycles." Flu epidemics were thought to come and go in periodic cycles, but it seemed that no two researchers could agree on precisely what the relevant time periods were nor which of them to utilize for purposes of estimating when—or if—the next major epidemic would occur: opinions ranged from three to ten to forty to ninety years, leaving the flu-epidemic prediction business somewhere between tea-leaf-reading and thoroughbred-racing perfecta analysis.

On the other hand, influenza was highly contagious—that

much was known for sure. You could pick up the virus from doorknobs, from an infected person's sneezing in a crowded room, et cetera—and the worst flu strains left heaps of dead people in their wake. Their unpredictability on the one hand coupled with their high infectiousness and occasional extreme virulence on the other gave public health officials max headaches when it came to protecting the community from flu viruses.

By the time of the Fort Dix case, indeed, many researchers were of the opinion that the world was long overdue for a major flu event, and by sheer coincidence, on February 13, the day before Sencer's emergency meeting, the *New York Times* had run an op-ed piece predicting that another influenza pandemic was on its way soon. Written by Edwin Kilbourne, a virologist at the Mt. Sinai School of Medicine in New York, the piece warned that "those concerned with public health had best plan without further delay for an imminent natural disaster."

Sencer's group, therefore, met in an atmosphere of some nervousness. Present at the meeting were Sencer and the usual CDC higher-ups, plus representatives from NIH, the FDA, the New Jersey Health Department, and the U.S. Army. With a national epidemic a theoretical possibility, their options ranged from keeping their eyes open for new cases to recommending a crash vaccination program for the coming flu season.

In favor of the first approach was the fact that the Fort Dix death had occurred in highly unusual circumstances. The victim, David Lewis, had been an otherwise healthy eighteen-year-old who'd come down with what seemed to be an ordinary case of the flu. He'd gone to the base clinic, where he was given the equally ordinary prescription of lots of fluids and bed rest. There was an upcoming five-mile nighttime training hike, however, and David Lewis, being an exceptionally gung ho trainee, was not about to be daunted by a few sniffles, doctor's orders or not. And so, against medical advice, he went out in the subzero windchills and heavy snow and ice and he slogged five miles through the dark with a fifty-pound pack on his back.

He collapsed during the march and was taken to the base hospital where, a few hours later, he died. Neither then nor at any point afterward had it been possible to say for sure what killed him: the flu, the hike, or a fatal combination of the two. These circumstances suggested a policy of great restraint when it came to drawing conclusions and taking action because, for one thing, the case was hardly typical. Far more important than that, however, was the fact that this was only a single case. "From one case—Private Lewis—you learn nothing," said Harvey Fineberg, dean of the Harvard School of Public Health, much later. For those reasons, the CDC group as a whole took the more cautious route and recommended only increased surveillance for new cases of swine flu; both Sencer himself and the Army's Philip Russell, however, were in favor of an immediate vaccine development program.

The CDC announced the Fort Dix swine flu death at a news conference the following week before publishing the test results and its formal recommendations in its journal of record, *Morbidity and Mortality Weekly Report*. At that point, though, the death took on a life of its own, as newspaper headlines like "Killer Flu Hits Military" set the stage for major hysteria, not on the part of the public, which looked upon the flu as a mere cold, but on the part of public health service officials and, worst of all, politicians. No matter how slight or even illusory the threat, politicians were always of the mind that "something's got to be done."

Soon, after several more emergency meetings, phone calls, private huddles, and hallway encounters, the CDC's initially cautious wait-and-see approach had escalated into the more reckless something's-got-to-be-done philosophy, even though very little data had arrived in the interim that made the prospect of an epidemic any more likely than it had been initially. Although there were some new cases of swine flu on the Fort

Dix base, there was still just the one known death from the disease, which meant that the variety going around was probably not identical to the highly lethal 1918 strain after all.

Nevertheless, by the end of a seven-hour marathon emergency CDC meeting on March 10, it looked as if the mass-vaccination alternative had prevailed. Dave Sencer, at the end of the meeting, had actually said, punningly, "It looks as if we'll have to go the whole hog."

There were, of course, some strong dissenters, people who regarded swine flu as "more of a curiosity than a threat," in the words of Walter Dowdle, head of the CDC's virology section. "I couldn't believe the decisions that had been made," he said later. "One or two people could sway the whole group. It was a marvel to see how this happened."

A couple of days after the March 10 meeting, Sencer had produced an "Action Memorandum" in which he described the crash vaccination program as one in which a new vaccine would be invented, mass-produced, distributed, and then administered to every last man, woman, and child in the country, some 196 million doses, all in the space of about seven or eight months. The price tag for all this was to be $134 million.

Sencer's memorandum worked its way up through the ranks until it reached the desk of Forrest David Mathews, the Secretary of Health, Education and Welfare. Mathews, in turn, sent an appropriations request to the Office of Management and Budget, together with a memo of his own that said: "There is evidence there will be a major flu epidemic this coming fall. The indication is that we will see a return of the 1918 flu virus that is the most virulent form of the flu. In 1918 a half million people died. The projections are that this virus will kill one million Americans in 1976."

So in the four-week period between the Valentine's Day meeting on February 14 and Mathews's budget-request memo of March 15, the isolated death of a sick Army recruit on a midnight hike in ice and snow had been converted into "pro-

171

jections" of a million dead Americans. Sencer's proposal now went to Gerald R. Ford, the president, who called a meeting of his own at the White House. It was attended by the cream of American medicine, including, in the words of one cynic, "the two most famous vaccinologists in the world," Jonas Salk and Albert Sabin. Having heard no opposition from any of them, the president that night went on national television to ask that $135 million be spent "to inoculate every man, woman, and child in the United States."

There now ensued "an almost unseemly race" in Congress, according to Arthur Silverstein, an aide to Senator Kennedy, to approve the spending bill, which was signed into law by the president in a televised ceremony on April 15. But the resulting program had a few imperfections of its own, one of which was that in field trials the vaccine worked poorly or not at all on children or younger adults, the very population whose lack of antibodies to the 1918 virus placed them at greatest risk for contracting the disease if exposed to the same pathogen. One company, Parke-Davis, manufactured 2 million doses against the wrong influenza strain.

Much worse than that, however, was that the vaccine was lethal to some who received it, people who probably would not have died had they not been vaccinated. Any vaccine produced occasional side effects—different people would have allergic reactions of greater or less severity—and this was especially true of a vaccine produced in a rush and then perhaps inadequately tested before use. The swine flu vaccine, it now turned out, caused Guillain-Barré syndrome, a rare wasting neurological disease in which, at the end of it, people looked like concentration camp victims, their limbs were that thin and emaciated. The Guillain-Barré disease was found in hundreds of people who received injections, fifty-eight of whom died. By December 16, in view of the problem, David Sencer called for an end to the mass vaccination program. It was never resumed.

In fact, it had not been needed in the first place because the swine flu virus never actually appeared that fall. According to Larry Schonberger, the CDC epidemiologist who'd first spotted the Guillain-Barré connection, it was clear by October 1, when vaccinations began, that chances were roughly 98 percent that the virus would never show up at all, and in fact it did not. The swine flu virus had disappeared from the United States long before the vaccination campaign began, and the fall of 1976, according to a later issue of *Morbidity and Mortality Weekly Report,* was an unusually disease-free period, with virtually no influenza of any type whatsoever, anywhere in North America.

The final tally of the whole exercise was: Known or suspected deaths due to swine flu: one, Pvt. David Lewis. Known or suspected deaths due to Guillain-Barré syndrome among those who had been vaccinated: fifty-eight. By 1993, more than four thousand claims had been filed against the U.S. government for Guillain-Barré syndrome caused by the swine flu vaccine, and more than $93 million had been paid out in damages.

The swine flu incident was a low point in the history of the CDC. Still, some of those involved would do essentially the same thing over again, Larry Schonberger, for one. "Look, mistakes were made, no doubt about that," he said in 1996, some twenty years after the incident. "And we now know that the military was a unique environment that encouraged spread of the flu. But we're talking about potentially saving the lives of thousands of people, and that can't be dismissed."

Walter Dowdle, by contrast, was a skeptic at the time, and he, too, had not appreciably changed his views. "I'd begin with the same alert phase," he said, "but then I'd have checkpoints along the way. You've got to monitor events to see if the program is still needed."

The truth was that the virus that appeared at Fort Dix in 1976 was almost certainly not the same one that had struck in 1918. "Nobody in the lab thought so at the time," said

Dowdle. "Flu viruses are always changing and reassorting, and this one had sixty years to do that. The probability that it was the same virus as the 1918 influenza strain was just extremely remote."

The whole thing was a learning experience for all concerned, many of whom could see the justice of Alexander Langmuir's remark from a long time back, that "the epidemiologist must recognize that prediction of future epidemics is a hazardous business."

Working epidemiologists, at any rate, seemed to be more cautious about their predictions thereafter. In 1988, a dozen years after the Great Swine Flu Affair, there was another single and unusual case of swine flu when a pregnant woman died of the virus after contracting it from a diseased pig while she and her husband visited the pig barns at a Wisconsin county fair. Her husband contracted the virus, too, and the infection was also transmitted to a few health care workers who'd treated the wife. The woman gave birth to a healthy baby three days before she died, and so in this case, as in the 1976 Fort Dix episode, there was only a single and isolated death.

This time, however, there was no apocalyptic thinking, no crash program, no politicians, and no mass vaccinations. And this time, too, there was no epidemic.

The first order of business in Kikwit had been to stop the outbreak by interrupting the chain of transmission, and that had been accomplished almost at once. The second order of business had been to map out all the lines of transmission and trace them back to the source; that took a bit longer, but with the discovery of the Menga family, that part of the project was well under way. The CDC therefore went ahead with its third and final mission objective, which was to locate the reservoir of the Ebola virus, and so in early June, a so-called ecological study team was sent to Zaire, people whose job it would be to collect a Noah's ark of the different animal species in and around Kikwit and send a representative sampling of them back to the lab in Atlanta.

Head of the animal team was John Krebs, a tall, thin, bearded zoologist who had ample past experience in Africa: in the late 1970s he'd spent four years in Sierra Leone studying the movements and infection patterns of *Mastomys natalensis,* the rodent vector of Lassa virus. Still, traveling to Kikwit was in a class by itself, and flying in on Air Kasai's DC-3 made him feel as if he were traveling backward in time.

Waiting there at the airport to greet them was Pierre Rollin, who had an extreme case of the smiles because he was going home on the return flight. So John Krebs stood at the field and watched him leave, this man who was going back to the outside world, to a place that already seemed like a far-off universe.

The DC-3 had a turnaround time of an hour or so, and Krebs watched as some vacuum flasks were loaded aboard, stainless steel canisters containing human blood and tissue samples immersed in liquid nitrogen. Then some white boxes went aboard, with further specimens on dry ice. Finally Pierre Rollin himself walked up the ramp and disappeared into the plane, followed by others who were on their way *out.*

The plane's hatch was closed, its engines started up, and in its slow and stately fashion the shining metal bird turned and taxied away.

Well, this is it, buddy, John Krebs thought to himself. *You can't just call a cab now if you suddenly change your mind about this.*

The plane stopped at the edge of the runway—a reasonably emotional juncture for Krebs, a metaphysical moment, a dividing line—and then its engines roared and the great silver beast moved forward, sped past . . . lifted off . . . became small in the sky.

You are now definitely here, John Krebs decided.

*   *   *

The normal workday for the ecological team began about six in the morning, when the faucets started gushing out their sunup ration of river water. You took a quick shower, ate, jumped in the four-wheel drive, always a Toyota Land Cruiser of some vintage—the whole city seemed like an advertisement for Toyota—and then you and the local driver plus three or four other team members bumped and bounced your way into the forest.

The famous and deserted Pont Mwembe forest.

It took about an hour to get there, lurching over a road that started out paved, turned into dirt ruts, then ended up as a narrow path gradually fading into the jungle. It was the dry season, anyway, thank God for that much. Some days there'd be a downed tree across the road, blocking forward progress just a bit, until one or more of the local bushwhackers hacked out a detour around it with knives.

Finally you arrived at the site itself, at Gaspard Menga's charcoal pit. For the virus hunters who'd come to Kikwit, this was hallowed ground. Virologically speaking, it was the center of creation. It was a landmark spot like Trinity Site or Hiroshima, the locus of the primal and explosive event. It was virus ground zero.

At virus ground zero people took turns standing in Gaspard Menga's historic and immortal charcoal pit and getting their picture taken. Don Noah, a veterinarian, stood there in hat and shirtsleeves, his long pants and combat boots, and struck a pose for his informal portrait. He, for one, wasn't worried about getting Ebola; that was the last thing on his mind. *This* wasn't where you got Ebola; the *hospital* was where you got Ebola.

"That was the kind of the way we looked at it," Don Noah said later. "There's only been a few outbreaks of Ebola in known history, so we weren't too concerned about walking through the forest."

The fact was, *everybody* was walking through the forest. Contrary to predictions and diametrically counter to all the rumors, the place was overrun by humans, by Kikwit natives. They came out in droves, throngs, in a mass procession, and they'd been doing this forever, every single day of the week. You could hardly turn around out there in the forest without bumping into a native Kikwitian tramping about in bare feet or flip-flops, like at the beach, carrying wood sticks, manioc, jugs of water, or whatever else. Indeed, there were even people *living* in the forest, whole families who *resided* there.

"We thought the forest was going to be this desolate place, but Lord no!" said Don Noah. "The jungle was just *full* of people. They were making charcoal, farming, hunting. Kikwit depopulates during the day and everybody goes into the jungle. And then at night they all walk back."

"It was a forest full of people," said Tom Ksiazek. "If you stood on the main road, there was an exceptionally large number of people who were going out of Kikwit. It's a very strange situation, sort of a reverse commuter situation, where people were going out to the forest where they had these small plots, where some of them were making charcoal. If you went to the area where we were trapping, you'd see a dozen—or a couple dozen—people go by."

If Ebola was truly the revenge of the rain forest, then all those people ought to be dead. But they were in fact so healthy, so very well-conditioned and able-bodied, that a fifteen-mile fast walk into the Pont Mwembe forest was considered nothing at all. These people were the marathon runners of Central Africa.

There may have been fewer animals out there than you might have expected—there were no monkeys or chimps to be found in Pont Mwembe forest—but that was because the Kikwitians had already come out there and eaten them all.

So John Krebs and Don Noah and a succession of CDC and other animal trappers would come out there, too, like proper Kikwitians, except that they'd be driven there in Land Cruisers, and they'd spend their day out in the jungle. They'd set traps—live-capture traps, most of them—for animals the size of mice or rats. They'd set about two hundred of the things, baiting them with peanut butter or something of the sort, then leave them on the ground overnight. Next day there'd be an average catch of 10 percent or so, which meant that you'd now have twenty or thirty possibly Ebola-laden wild animals, most of them with sharp teeth, fangs, and claws, hip-hopping around in the traps, some of them screaming their lungs out. The object was to collect blood and tissue samples from these monsters without killing yourself in the process.

First thing you did, you got dressed in surgeon's gown or coveralls, shoe covers, two pairs of latex gloves, plus face masks and goggles—all this in high heat and humidity. Then with gloved hands you picked up the trap containing this furry, live thing, and if there was a breeze, you'd stand with your back to the wind so that the invisible Ebola particles, if any, that were coming up and off the beast would be blown away from instead of toward you, and at that point you'd anesthetize the animal. (People got jaded quickly enough and soon began holding some of the animals in their bare hands while dressed in street clothes. They'd cradle the beast, almost cuddle it, and show it to you as they would a kitten.)

If the trap was small enough, you could place it whole into a clear plastic bag containing gauze or cotton soaked with an inhalant anesthetic. But if the trap was too big for that, then you shook out the beast into the plastic bag, hoping to God it would be knocked cold before it chewed its way out. ("Technicians should take care to minimize inhaling anesthesia during these procedures," the official CDC guidelines said.)

A third method of knocking them out was by injection. "We do have some needles for injecting larger animals, or reptiles, with a different anesthetic," said John Krebs. "But when those needles are being used, we're all acutely aware that they are being used. Each one of us is reminding the other to be careful with the needle."

The animal would, finally, be asleep—in "anesthetic repose," they jokingly called it—and now you could take your blood sample or sacrifice the animal and take a tissue sample or whatever. For the latter procedure it was wise to wear a battery-powered respirator, a face mask that blew air out from any gaps so that no extraneous matter could come in.

"A secondary benefit of these respirators is that they keep the flies off your face," said Krebs. "That's quite important with the type of work that we're doing."

So you'd lay the dead brute flat on its back, make an incision with dissection scissors, and with sterile, blunt-end forceps you'd remove some or all of the relevant organs. Another member of the team would place the samples in labeled vials and immediately put them on ice, the start of the cold chain that would preserve them until they were finally thawed out back in Atlanta.

It was a teamwork operation, with people sitting around shaded worktables, all of them performing their own tasks. Since it was important to keep each sample pure and uncontaminated, sterility had to be maintained, which meant that everything had to be disinfected regularly: instruments, work surfaces, and even the traps, which had to be cleaned out and washed before the next use. Sometimes the whole process took a bit longer than expected, and in fact the very first day they went into the jungle, Krebs and his crew were still out in the field as the sun was going down.

"When the sun falls in Africa, it falls fairly quickly and so it was getting quite dark," he recalled later. "And we didn't have our flashlights with us because we didn't anticipate being out there that long.

"We got back all right and we were never really in danger," he added. "Still, we had a little bit of a rapid heartbeat that first night."

* * *

179

Back in Atlanta, the Kikwit samples went into freezers where they waited in silence for their turn to be tested. The number of specimens soon reached into the thousands, which made for a rather long wait. In the past, however, some of those long waits had eventually paid off.

In 1977, almost twelve years after they'd been entombed in freezers at the Lab of Last Resort in Atlanta, the microbes responsible for the St. Elizabeth's Hospital pneumonia epidemic in July of 1965 were defrosted and resurrected. And so were the specimens that dated back to July of 1968, when ninety-five out of one hundred employees of the Pontiac, Michigan, health department called in sick with an unexplained respiratory disease. Those same anonymous microbes were again on the loose; this time, however, the CDC's lab men were able to put a name and number to the beast.

It was the middle of summer again—it was July, in fact, just like before—and the microbes had chosen to invade a single building, as had been their previous modus operandi. They'd made their comeback in Philadelphia, at the Bellevue-Stratford Hotel, where they'd run wild through a bunch of Legionnaires, American war veterans, attending the state convention. By August 2, 1976, there were one hundred and fifty cases of the pneumonia-like illness, and twenty people, most of them elderly men, had died. It would start with something like flu symptoms, then escalate into high fever, chills, muscle aches, and headaches. Dry cough, gastrointestinal pain, and diarrhea were also common. In a weird bit of coincidental timing, this was happening during the precise same year and month that another unnamed pathogen was making its first known appearance in the town of Yambuku, Zaire, not far from the river Ebola. The symptomatology of the two diseases were much alike, except for the lack of hemorrhaging among the Legionnaires, who seemed to be the sole targets of the disease in Philadelphia.

Pretty soon everybody in the country had seen televised footage of flag-draped coffins being lowered into the ground, antique soldiers marching through city streets, and white-coated laboratory people shaking their heads and saying, "We don't know yet what's causing these deaths," and so on. Even some normally staid and sober medical journals were running stories about "the explosive outbreak," the "mysterious and terrifying" disease, and the like.

Beyond that, some fairly outlandish rumors were going around about the cause of it all. After traces of nickel had been found in tissue samples taken from some of the first victims, the disease was attributed to nickel poisoning, and Jack Anderson, the Washington columnist—not a major medical writer, admittedly—published a story about a mad poisoner on the loose, a crazed killer who for unknown reasons had salted the hotel's air-conditioning ducts with a noxious dry-ice, nickel-carbonyl death potion. (The nickel deposits were actually post-mortem contamination, bits of the metal that had flaked off surgical instruments during autopsy.)

Magic even entered the picture when CDC epidemiologists—a total of twenty-five had been sent up there—learned that the hotel involved, the Bellevue-Stratford, had hosted a magicians convention just a week prior to the Legionnaires gathering. The CDC's David Heymann, who'd stay in the same hotel for the whole of the investigation, tracked down the head of the magicians union and grilled him about their having used any new-wave magic tricks involving smoke, steam, fumes, or whatever. But in fact they'd only been up to their same old magic, and so that, too, was a trail that led nowhere. People began to despair of ever finding the cause, and CDC's Bill Foege, at one point, said, "In five, ten, or twenty years from now when our technology is further advanced, we will find out what killed the Legionnaires."

All those wild rumors and morbid conclusions went the way of all flesh, however, when the infectious agent was finally

identified a few months later. What was killing the Legionnaires, it turned out, was not nickel poisoning or black magic
or Ebola or any other obscure virus; it was, instead, a type of
bacteria, one that had never before been recognized, although
it had probably been around from time immemorial, as it
thrived quite happily in all manner of commonplace environments such as mud puddles, creeks, and stagnant pools of
water. Indeed, when it was all over and done with, the CDC
would estimate that literally thousands of people had been
dying of the organism each year for decades, with the deaths
attributed to one or another variety of "pneumonia of unknown etiology."

The identification took five months of lab work—a long time,
but not a world record—for reasons that became entirely clear
after the fact. Two CDC scientists, Charles Shepard and Joe
McDade, had tested the Legionnaires samples for every imaginable infectious agent for several weeks in the late summer of
1976, but for all that work they had nothing much to show for
it. True, there'd been some puzzling results and false positives
and one thing and another, including, as Joe McDade later
remembered, "an extraneous rod-shaped organism" that
popped up every now and then on his microscope slides. He'd
first seen them in August, just a few weeks after the outbreak.

Those rod-shaped organisms were bacteria, but nobody saw
very many of them, and more important, nobody could manage
to culture them from the samples, and so everybody had pretty
much dismissed them from consideration. The agent, they concluded, had to be viral or rickettsial.

In Joe McDade's view, however, maybe they really *were* bacterial. Biological testing work, he knew, was not exactly cut-
and-dried; to grow a microbe you faced a bunch of choices:
you could use human tissues, animal tissues, chicken eggs,
various prepared culture media, smears, blots, et cetera, in addition to which you relied on a whole galloping variety of
stains, techniques, and esoteric lab gimmicks to produce re-

sults. It was unequal parts science and art, and in many cases the outcome depended as much on the skill of the investigator as on any inherent qualities of the microbe.

So during the Christmas holidays of 1976, at which time he had a few spare moments to run the tests again, Joe McDade, the junior man on the team, decided he'd have another little look-see. He removed a slide from the little wooden slide box on his desk, clipped it onto the focusable stage of the microscope, and peered down through the eyepiece. This time, for some reason, he saw *lots* of those "extraneous rod-shaped organisms," clumps of them, whole small colonies of the things. They hadn't multiplied in the interim, they'd been there beforehand, he'd just never looked at the right places on the slides. "It was like looking for a contact lens on a basketball court by crawling on your hands and knees with your eyes only four inches from the floor," he said later.

He repeated the process with other slides and saw even more of those tiny rods, so he tried to grow them out so that he'd have enough of the stuff to test against antibodies from the human victims. This time he was successful, and the result was a strong positive match with the Legionnaires' antibodies: this was the bacterium that had gone around in Philadelphia five months previously.

Then, from the fact that it wouldn't react with any other substance in the CDC's vast storehouse of diagnostic reagents, McDade and company concluded that it was a microbe that neither they nor anyone else had ever before put a name to. It was a newly recognized pathogen, a bacterium that they named *Legionella pneumophila*.

Now that they had it there in front of them, they remembered the unsolved St. Elizabeth's case, which had also involved people in a single building dying of unexplained pneumonia in the month of July. So they went back to the freezers, extracted the St. Elizabeth's samples from their eleven-year stay in frozen limbo, and thawed them out. As suspected, they contained *Legionella* bacteria.

The microbe must have been in the soil all along, then was stirred up by the earth-moving activity outside the St. Elizabeth's hospital ward and brought into the building on gusts of wind. Those had been the identical circumstances in the Pontiac fever case, and so a few days after the St. Elizabeth's discovery, they went back to the freezers a second time and pulled out the Pontiac fever samples. They, too, were positive for *Legionella*.

The puzzling part of it all was why, if it were truly the same agent as in the St. Elizabeth's case and in Philadelphia, it hadn't killed anyone in Michigan. Ninety-five people had gotten sick in Pontiac, but there'd not been a single fatality, and in fact only one person was even hospitalized.

"It might be a *forme fruste,* an incomplete or mild form of a disease, one that spontaneously stops before its normal course is run," said Michael Gregg, a physician who'd been on the original Pontiac fever investigation team. "It might be caused by a dead organism, one that's encapsulated, contorted, or compressed, an essentially dead form of the bacterium, whereas in Legionnaires' disease proper the organism is still alive. So they might be two clinically different diseases caused by two forms of the same organism."

McDade and his colleagues now had an explanation for why it had taken them so long to isolate and identify the bug. The organism, they'd discovered, was rather eccentric, since it refused to grow in the same culture media that most other bacteria seemed to flourish in. This microbe actually preferred total darkness—the insides of water pipes, cooling ducts, and the like—and so when it couldn't be grown in the conventional way, the researchers concluded that it must instead be a virus, and so they tried to grow it like a virus. That meant adding antibiotics to the growth medium, to kill off any stray bacteria that might interfere with growth of the virus, but those same antibiotics killed off the very microbe that had been responsible for the outbreak.

They'd finally figured it all out, and in identifying the *Legionella* agent, McDade, Shepard, and their CDC colleagues solved a whole slew of medical mysteries, one of which had gone back more than a decade, plus which they'd learned something new about testing procedures for unknown pathogens—all in one fell swoop. In the annals of infectious diseases research, this was progress.

The Rocky Mountain spotted fever accident, where two died, was not progress, but it did have a positive effect in that it motivated the CDC to think about building a new laboratory facility. If the world's worst pathogens were inevitably going to wind up at the Lab of Last Resort, then the place could at least have a separate and freestanding structure whose major purpose was to house those agents in reasonable safety.

Karl Johnson's hand-me-down lab from the NIH—the "thing"—safe and secure though it had always been in his hands, "was a makeshift thing," he said. "It was also tiny in a world where a new Level 4 agent seemed to crop up each year."

But the old agents presented a considerable threat all by themselves, even those, such as smallpox, that had otherwise been wiped out of existence. One of the final concerns of the global smallpox eradication team, in fact, had been to enumerate all the possible ways in which the smallpox virus could come back out into the world at large. This was by no means a paranoid worry, as became clear after they'd put together the list. For example, the disease could emerge from an as-yet-unidentified animal host. It could come from deliberate release on the part of some individual or agency who for reasons of its own had stored away samples of the virus. Most worrisome of all was the prospect that the smallpox virus could accidentally escape from an approved and certified storage facility—a biological research lab.

In 1978, several months after the disease had been eradicated from the world, that actually happened when a photographer who worked for the Medical School at the University of Birmingham, in England, contracted smallpox and died from the disease. This was a major scandal: biological labs were supposed to be safe, but she'd gotten the disease from the university's smallpox lab one floor below her own office.

That lab, supposedly, was physically sealed off from the rest of the building: the tiny eight-by-eight-foot closed chamber was situated in one corner of the bigger animal-pox room and protected by means of negative air pressure. In addition, all sorts of policies and safeguards were officially in place to prevent any accidental escapes and infections: all smallpox work was to be carried out within the biological safety cabinet inside the smaller room; laboratory gowns were to be autoclaved immediately after use; used pipettes were to be completely submerged in disinfectant and then discarded; all lab personnel, and anyone else remotely connected with the place, were to be regularly vaccinated against smallpox.

But all those policies and procedures were routinely ignored: not all smallpox work was carried out in the safety cabinet, and in fact some of it was done in the open spaces of the animal-pox room; lab gowns were autoclaved weekly instead of daily; contaminated pipettes often overflowed the discard bucket; and so on and so forth.

As for the alleged hermetic isolation of the lab, that, too, was largely a grand illusion. Air flowed out of the smallpox room every time the door was opened: it drifted into the animal-pox room, into the seminar room next door, and out into the adjoining corridor. Worst of all, air from the lab seeped into service ducts that connected the animal-pox room to the photographer's office on the floor above. That was enough of a route for the virus, which could float around invisibly on a current of air. As would happen repeatedly in the history of infectious diseases, inert viruses were helped along by the negligent behavior of human beings.

The lessons from all this were clear enough. There was no ironclad protection against human error and fatal lapses of safety procedures, and the lab couldn't be built whose best features weren't defeatable by people. But if no lab could be totally fail-safe, one could at least be constructed that was airtight and optimally error-resistant, which was the idea behind CDC's new maximum containment lab.

It would be a pristine and autonomous place, a separate building all by itself—access-restricted, monitored by closed-circuit, remote-controlled television cameras, safeguarded and impregnable—where highly trained, space-suited lab creatures worked in an artificial, sealed, and sterile environment. It would be like a submarine or space capsule, only firmly planted on the ground in Atlanta. Unauthorized people could not get in. Unauthorized microbes could not get out. It would be its own little self-contained universe, the most hygienic and healthiest place in the cosmos.

Which is just about what it became. It took only a decade or so from the very first glimmerings to the actual implementation—not so bad for government work. But when Building 15, the Viral and Rickettsial Diseases Laboratory, finally opened in 1988, well, it was a place apart and a marvel to behold. It was like the space station in *2001: A Space Odyssey*, only it didn't rotate. It had eleven separate Level 3 hot suites, all of them bright, pleasant, and surgically clean. The Level 4 labs—the maximum containment suites—were off in their own separate wing, and you entered them in space suits and you went through air locks, just exactly like an astronaut.

No two ways about it, CDC's Building 15 was the promised land. It was the Grand Hyatt Regency of the laboratory kingdom. It just did not get any better than this.

10 The "Emerging Diseases" Irony

Like the FBI or Scotland Yard, the CDC was in the business of crime detection. Tracing a bunch of deaths back to a biological killer was medical detective work in the most literal sense, a species of true crime. That the perpetrators were tiny and invisible only made the job more of a challenge than ordinary police work, which was fairly straightforward in comparison. The homicide detective trafficked in lists of suspects, physical evidence, eyewitness testimony, and alibis. You knew you had the guilty party when one or more persons could be proved to have means, opportunity, and motive and could be linked to the crime by physical evidence in the form of fingerprints, bloodstains, footprints, and the like. But microbes, too, had means and opportunity, and even a motive for their crimes against humanity. The means by which they killed was through infection, which was to say by physically entering the body and taking over one or more internal organs, often replicating within them. They had opportunity whenever there was contact between microbe and victim, and in the case of airborne infections, that contact could occur by air. The motive, finally, was sheer survival, for this was how microbes made a living, by finding congenial new biological hosts to attack.

Investigating a microbial crime, therefore, meant visiting the site and sifting for evidence. Sometimes the process imitated detective fiction a bit too closely for comfort.

In the canonical scene of a Tony Hillerman mystery, Jim Chee, a Navajo Indian and officer of the Navajo Tribal Police of Window Rock, Arizona, drives to the victim's home, enters it, and searches the place for clues. Often enough this is a mobile home, a rusted trailer on the red mesa, where some backwoods Indian lived peaceably and alone until his life ended suddenly in a blaze of violence. Later there's an autopsy, a series of routine interrogations of relatives and friends, and sometimes even a reconstruction of the crime. At some point, the authorities visit the tribal elders, who divulge precious morsels of relevant lore from out of their indigenous oral tradition.

There are car chases and wild-goose chases all over the Four Corners region, plus a midnight ride through Monument Valley, a fabulous desert landscape strewn with rocks, buttes, and lone vertical monoliths. Predictably, there are false leads, ploys, and diversions, together with one or more additional deaths, before the forces of justice—almost but not quite stopped in their tracks by ancient tribal customs and taboos—identify and capture the guilty party.

And so it was in real life when on May 14, 1993, Merrill Bahe, a Navajo boy aged nineteen and a marathon runner in the peak of health, died suddenly and mysteriously, gasping for breath, while riding in a car barreling through the desert near Gallup, New Mexico, about twenty miles east of Window Rock.

Merrill Bahe lived in a trailer.

His fiancée, who lived there with him, had died equally without warning a few days earlier, gulping for air in the same manner. He'd been on his way to her funeral, in fact, when he was taken ill.

A few days after these events, an investigator from the Indian Health Service in Albuquerque, himself a Cherokee Indian, drove out to the trailer, entered it, and searched the place for clues.

His name was Jim Cheek.

When he opened the trailer door and stepped in, Jim Cheek faced the usual detritus of human existence: clothing, dirty dishes, garbage. He took up various samples for later analysis. He also found an abnormally large quantity of mouse droppings, and although he was unprotected by gloves, face mask, or goggles, he collected samples of the droppings, too, and brought them back to the lab.

It was the start of an investigation into a series of unexpected and puzzling deaths in the Four Corners region. Twelve people would die with similar symptoms within the next few weeks, many of them Native Americans living within the borders of the Navajo Indian Reservation, an enormous twenty-thousand-square-mile area about twice the size of Massachusetts.

And then the epidemic started spreading. New cases cropped up in Texas, California, Oregon, and elsewhere, and mysteriously, some of the new victims were also Native Americans.

There was a fourteen-year-old boy in Fort Totten, North Dakota, a member of the Devils Lake Sioux Tribe, which was located about a hundred miles west of Grand Forks, and nowhere near Four Corners. When he showed up at a clinic in the area, the boy had a temperature of 101° F, a heart rate of 120 beats per minute, and rales—abnormal breathing sounds from the lungs. He was diagnosed with pneumonia, given a variety of drugs, and sent home.

He was back again that same afternoon, however, with an

even higher temperature and pulse rate, at which time he was given an intramuscular injection of antibiotic.

The next day he showed some improvement, but on the following morning—day three of his illness—he collapsed at home and was brought to the local emergency room. According to the published report on the case: "He was noted to be pale, with dry mucous membranes; bluish lips, fingers, and nails . . . He was placed on a non-rebreathing oxygen face mask with an oxygen saturation of 86%. . . . Within 20 minutes of arrival he became asystolic [without heartbeat] and was successfully resuscitated. However, forty-five minutes later, he developed a nonperfusing bradyarrythmia [abnormally slow heartbeat] and attempts to resuscitate him were unsuccessful."

The disease, whatever it was, caused an unnaturally fast decline and fall, and it seemed to have abnormal inclination for Native Americans, as if this truly were some nightmare contagion that for unknown reasons zeroed in upon the American Indian. The Navajo themselves, who regarded untimely deaths as a punishment for bad living, wondered if the illness was not retribution for their having embraced such white man's evils as fast food, MTV, and video games. If so, the cure for what ailed them would not lie within the purview of science. "Western medicine has its limitations," said Navajo president Peterson Zah.

Even so, within three weeks the CDC identified the offending microbe as hantavirus and in two more weeks had found the animal reservoir, the deer mouse. Shortly after that they'd put together a set of guidelines for reducing the risk of exposure to the microbe and had published them in *Morbidity and Mortality Weekly Report*, which was routinely sent to public health officials all across the country.

The Four Corners episode proved to be a landmark case for the CDC. The operation ran in record time and went off without a hitch, and the CDC emerged from it looking like a perfectly designed bureaucratic machine successfully doing its job in silence, which in this case it was.

The irony was that the CDC's increasing successes identifying pathogens were looked upon as ominous and threatening, as foreshadowing uncontrolled outbreaks of "new" and "emerging" diseases. Most of the microbes and diseases that the CDC dealt with, however, were not "new" by any standard. Certainly Legionnaires' disease was not: it had "emerged" a long time ago, well before the Legionnaires themselves began falling ill in Philadelphia in 1976, before the county health workers started calling in sick in Pontiac, Michigan, in 1968, and before the St. Elizabeth's patients started dying of pneumonia in July of 1965. The affliction, so far as anyone could tell, went well back into the far reaches of disease history, as did the microbes that caused it. "The bacterium was new only in the sense that it was unfamiliar to laboratory workers," said Joe McDade of the *Legionella* microbe. "The identical bacterium had been isolated in 1947 from a guinea pig inoculated with blood from a patient who had a febrile respiratory illness."

Prior cases of the disease were hard to prove mainly because of the lack of earlier blood or tissue samples that could be submitted to tests. Later cases, however, appeared like clockwork, and soon Legionnaires' disease was "emerging" all over the world.

It was "emerging," however, only in the sense that the disease detectives now had the rapid diagnostic tests, plus lab techniques, instruments, and vast storehouses of reagents, that permitted them to recognize it easily enough when and where it occurred. The availability of these standardized tests, and the tremendous diagnostic power represented by the store of reagents, contributed to the false impression that new diseases were springing up all over the world, like shopping centers, whereas in reality the main thing that was new was the ease and speed with which these diseases could now be identified.

The hantaviruses, for example, were an ancient species of

microbe, some of which were thought to have caused outbreaks as far back as A.D. 960. The name itself—originally
"Hantaan virus"—was relatively new, coined in 1978 for an
outbreak near the Hantaan River in Korea in which 121 American soldiers died among the 2,000 who were stationed in the
area. There had been several earlier epidemics of closely related diseases, however, including one in Sweden in 1934, and
others in the Soviet Union between 1913 and 1935. The syndrome was common in northwestern Europe, and between
1977 and 1995 some 505 cases had been recorded in north-
eastern France alone.

"What are commonly termed emerging pathogens are not
really new," said Bernard Le Guenno, the Pasteur Institute
virologist. "What appear to be novel viruses are generally viruses that have existed for millions of years."

The rise of "emerging diseases," therefore, was largely an
illusion fostered by CDC's own rapidly increasing success at
unraveling previously unsolved medical mysteries and discovering previously undetected microbial crimes. The irony of
it all was that the better the CDC got at identifying the pathogens that caused age-old but hitherto unrecognized diseases,
the more it looked as if scads of trailblazing new microbes were
out there amassing themselves for attack, gathering their forces,
and preparing to bring us "the coming plague."

The more successful the CDC became, in other words, the
more diseased the world looked.

But it wasn't. By almost every measure, the world's peoples
were getting steadily healthier: average life expectancy was on
the increase, worldwide, among all races; infant and child mortality rates were consistently declining, in both developed and
developing countries; the world's population routinely grew,
and indeed it had grown fastest in Africa itself, for at least
the last twenty years. Outbreaks of *health*, however, were not
considered "news."

*   *   *

By the time Gary Maupin arrived in Kikwit, the epidemic was distinctly winding down. At the end of June there were only one or two new Ebola deaths per day, and sometimes none at all—nothing like the ten or twelve daily fatalities that Pierre and Philippe had had to contend with at the height of the crisis.

Gary Maupin was an entomologist—a bug specialist. He was from Colorado, where he'd worked the last twenty-four years, the whole time at the CDC's outpost in Fort Collins. He'd graduated from Colorado State in 1970 with a master's degree in zoology and medical entomology and then about three days later joined the CDC, where he'd been ever since. One of the diseases he dealt with out there was bubonic plague.

Bubonic plague was one of the success stories of Western medicine. The Black Death had killed about one-third of the European population, some 20 to 30 million people, back in the 1300s when it ripped through the Continent, but in the twentieth century the disease had been almost totally eradicated from both Europe and the United States. Still, it had never been eradicated entirely, and the American Southwest averaged ten cases of bubonic plague per year. "In 1983 there were forty cases, which is the high in recent times," said Gary Maupin.

The disease was caused by bacteria harbored in the intestinal tracts of fleas, which were in turn carried by various rodents, mainly rats and mice but also by rabbits, squirrels, prairie dogs, and marmots, and even domestic dogs and cats. Maupin once investigated a case in Cheyenne, Wyoming, in which a veterinary technician had gotten the disease from a house cat that had been brought to the clinic with swollen maxillary lymph nodes—a sign of bubonic plague. The cat was having a hard time breathing, and the technician was face-to-face with the animal, which was trying to clear its air passages, when suddenly the animal coughed in her face, and shortly she, too, had bubonic plague.

The disease was treated with antibiotics and she recovered from the infection without any problem. Later Maupin traced the microbe back to ground squirrels on the cat owner's five-acre property east of Cheyenne. In his years with the CDC, Maupin had been all over the Wild West and had trapped countless fleas, ticks, and other insects in all sorts of urban and rural environments, but nothing that he'd seen in all his years exactly prepared him for what he saw in Kikwit.

The assorted bugs in the Hôtel Kwilu, where he'd stayed for a few nights before transferring over to George's house, were not the problem. He was, after all, an entomologist.

"Didn't bother me at all," Gary Maupin said. "I was a little tired of the mosquito bites on the ears at night."

But he later transferred over to George's house, where he slept under mosquito netting, after which there were no more bites. What took some getting used to at George's house were the morning traffic jams.

"There were I don't know how many different activities going on at that point," he said. "Mammal trapping, work at the hospital, work at the clinic, entomological teams. Everybody had a different destination and different duties and activities during the day. It would take a little time and patience in the morning to get everybody where they needed to go, simply because of not enough vehicles and so many people."

The madding crowds did not thin out significantly even in the forest, the famous and deserted Pont Mwembe forest, where there were "hundreds of people! Gathering wood, harvesting papaya, banana, manioc, manioc roots, tubers, manioc leaves, anything that's edible."

The other surprise was the relative lack of insects at virus ground zero, Gaspard Menga's charcoal pit.

"We traveled that whole area where the supposed index case centered his activities: the charcoal pit and the little farming plot, looking for ticks or any ectoparasites that could be involved in transmission of the disease. We looked in every hole in the ground. We dragged one-meter-square pieces of cloth over the surface of the ground looking for questing ticks, especially along trails and any open areas where there's human activity, such as the farm-plot edge. We looked in some tree holes, basically in downed trees because we didn't have tree-climbing equipment to get way up. But we didn't find any ticks at all. Everything was negative."

In fact the only ticks he ever saw came from the wild and domestic animal population in and around Kikwit. The ecological team sent word out that they were looking for bugs, that they'd actually pay for ticks—a nickel for twenty, some such rate—after which they got as many as they could handle.

"When the local population found out we were paying for bugs," said Don Noah, "they'd bring their dogs by and sell us the ticks off the dog. We got two hundred ticks off of one dog."

A pangolin—a scaly anteater—had twenty-two ticks on it. A cane rat had half a dozen, a civet cat had two more, et cetera.

Then there were the bedbugs: small, oval-shaped, reddish brown insects that lived by sucking human blood. Conceivably, bedbugs were an Ebola vector. The population of Kikwit, anyway, had learned by this time not to sleep in the same bed as an Ebola victim: you didn't want to share that person's bedbugs, which, in the homes of Kikwit, were as common as flies.

The homes tended to be made out of concrete blocks or mud and wattle. Inside there would be kids, animals, sometimes chickens roosting in one of the rooms. There'd be some wooden furniture—table, chairs, and one or more beds. They were typically wood-frame beds with crosswise slats with a bamboo or palm-leaf mat laid on top, and maybe a sheet or blanket covering the mat. During the day the bedbugs lived in the cracks and crevices in the wooden bedframes; at night they'd crawl out and feed on the sleeping people.

So Gary Maupin and his crew now went inside people's homes looking for bedbugs. It was usually pretty dark in the homes; the bedbugs, though, were easy to find.

"All you had to do was take the bedframes, the wooden bedframes inside these houses, out into the sunlight and literally pick the bedbugs off the bedframe," he said. "Sometimes we just collected them until we got tired because there was no way to collect all of them. We asked the team members to please collect at least a hundred bedbugs from each household, and very seldom did they get fewer than that."

In the end, Gary Maupin's entomological team took nine thousand bedbugs from homes in Kikwit.

The occasion for all the activity in Kikwit was the Ebola virus itself, a small molecular structure that was in fact only a bunch of chemicals strung together in a long line. On the other hand, that was what most everything in the world was, bunches of chemicals clumped together, and every day the average person met up with countless trillions of such small molecular structures, and none of them caused any problem. The very air itself was full of them, full of chemical molecules from smoke to smog, floating proteins, tiny crystals, metal flakes, oil droplets, bits of silicon, rock chips, flying vitamins, pieces of cotton—incredible amounts of molecular flotsam and jetsam. Beyond that the air was full of the most hideous microbiological monsters imaginable: bacteria, yeasts, pollen grains, spores, funguses, rusts, tiny bugs. You breathed that stuff in and out every minute of every day, and you never even gave it a thought.

So what was so special about the Ebola molecule? It was far more complex than a metal flake but far simpler than a pollen grain, which was, sizewise, bigger than even the largest virus. Pollen grains, indeed, were often infected by viruses of their own. The mystery, then, was how and why this little line of chemicals had the ability to convert a person's internal organs to slime shortly after entering the body.

That mystery, too, was under investigation at the CDC, and

197

in the spring of 1995, at about the time the Ebola virus was breaking out in Kikwit, four of the main players of the drama, C. J. Peters, Anthony Sanchez, Pierre Rollin, and Tom Ksiazek, were writing a joint scientific paper about the filoviruses, Marburg and Ebola. (Fred Murphy, who'd done much of the original Marburg work back in the late 1960s, was the fifth coauthor.) The paper was entitled "Filoviridae: Marburg and Ebola Viruses" and would appear in the 1996 edition of the bible of virological knowledge, *Fields Virology*, edited by Bernard Fields, of Harvard.

For a work that purported to summarize the state of the art, the amazing part of it was the number of things that were still unknown. "We still do not know how filoviruses are maintained in nature," the authors said. "It has generally been possible to identify an index human case or index group of imported nonhuman primates, but the source of their infection has remained an enigma. . . .

"The mode of entry of Marburg and Ebola viruses into cells remains unknown. . . .

"The origins of the pathophysiologic changes that make Marburg and Ebola virus infections of humans so devastating are still not understood. . . .

"In fatal filovirus infections, the host dies with high viremia and generally no evidence of an immune response. . . . The reason for the failure to respond is unknown. . . .

"In humans, monkeys, and guinea pigs, the mechanism of ,recovery from filovirus infection is unknown. . . .

"The origin in nature and the natural history of Marburg and Ebola viruses remain a mystery."

In other words, nobody knew what the natural reservoir of the viruses was, exactly how these viruses infiltrated the cells they attacked, why they were as lethal as they were, why in most cases the immune system failed to offer protection against them, and why, in the cases where it *did* offer protection, it was successful in doing so.

That was a lot to be in the dark about. On the other hand, what was known about these viruses was quite astonishing in its own right. The main difference between a molecule of Ebola and a bit of random substance like a metal flake or an oil drop was that the Ebola molecule consisted of a code. Its chemical components were arranged in precise groupings of nucleotides, the building blocks of RNA and DNA. A given discrete sequence of nucleotides, or bases, made up a gene, and a given gene coded for a certain protein, which was one of the things that a complete virus molecule was made up of. The complete order of these nucleotides was rigorously determined and absolutely unique: there was no other combination of those exact base sequences anywhere else in nature.

How those sequences worked upon human cells was the preserve of the CDC's Anthony Sanchez, one of the few people in the world to have written a Ph.D. dissertation on the Marburg virus.

Sanchez was a second-generation Mexican-American who grew up in Safford, Arizona, a small farming community in the southeast part of the state. He started out as a microbiologist and worked for a while as a clinician for the Indian Health Service in Phoenix, doing diagnostic tests on the bodily fluids and tissues of sick patients. That kind of work held a finite interest for Sanchez, and after a while he decided that he was really cut out to be a researcher, finding out why these tiny molecular objects behaved in the various ways they did. One thing led to another, and by 1981, at the age of twenty-eight, he was in Atlanta and working at the CDC as a research microbiologist in the Special Pathogens Branch. Simultaneously, he went for his Ph.D. in molecular genetics from Georgia State. He liked to work with the filoviruses—Marburg and Ebola— because they were so benign and tractable, at least in the test tube.

"From the beginning, I had always been somewhat enchanted by the filoviruses," he said, "by their ability to grow to very high concentrations, to be easily purified, and just be very cooperative agents in terms of doing what you set out to do. Also, their reputation as being extremely pathogenic was a little bit enticing, and so I've been working on these agents for the last twelve years."

Among other things, he discovered and published the nucleotide sequences of the first six genes of the 1976 Ebola-Zaire subtype, which meant that he established the precise combination of molecular bases that made up each of those six component parts of the virus. (The Ebola virus had a total of seven genes; a group of Russian scientists sequenced the seventh gene.) The entire genome—the complete set of bases contained in all the genes—was rather long, at least for a virus. Genome lengths were measured in kilobases (thousands of bases), and whereas some viruses, such as rabies, were twelve kilobases in length, the filoviruses were approximately nineteen kilobases long, made up of nineteen thousand chemical subunits, meaning that a fairly large amount of information was packed into a single molecule of Ebola virus.

Sanchez experimented with the individual genes of the virus, separating them out from the rest of the genome and inserting them into various cell cultures. This was a standard molecular-biology research technique because it allowed you to discover the function of a given gene: you inserted the gene into a culture of known cell types, thereby causing the cells to synthesize whatever it was the gene coded for.

One of the Ebola virus's genes encoded the instructions for making the outer surface of the virus particle, its so-called outer envelope. The outer envelope was the part of the virus that made physical contact with a host cell. The envelope bristled with spiky projections and protrusions, and these surface spikes fitted into complementary molecular structures on the cell's surface.

"This surface spike attaches to molecules on the cell and allows the virus to gain entry into it, so they're very important structures," said Sanchez. "We found something very bizarre going on with the gene that encodes the spike structure."

The "very bizarre" activity that Sanchez discovered was that one sequence of molecular instructions was performing a sort of double duty: it simultaneously encoded two different gene products. That practically violated the rules of molecular biology, which stated that one gene normally made one protein, just as one part of a computer program normally gave you one output. The glycoprotein gene of the Ebola virus, however, had *two distinct products,* one being the system of spiky projections on the virus's outer envelope, the other being a liquid, a secreted or soluble glycoprotein, that never became part of the virus at all. Instead, it floated away from the virus and migrated off to parts unknown.

Sanchez also discovered exactly how it was that the Ebola virus's genetic code managed to accomplish this feat of double-duty molecular coding. He found that the same piece of code was being read and copied twice, once before and once after "an editing or frameshifting event." The code was read once starting at a given point, then it was read again starting at another point that differed by one nucleotide from the first. That new starting point yielded a whole new molecular message.

"The virus has made the best use of this limited sequence," said Sanchez. "It's using two frames to generate two proteins. So the dynamics of the thing are very intriguing."

This bit of molecular magic was so wholly improbable, so truly subtle and clever, that it was hard to believe anything so small and lowly as a virus could accomplish it. But the Ebola virus was clever enough, and it did. The question was, why did the virus go through all the trouble? Why did it turn out this extra gene product, a secreted glycoprotein that floated off and away and never even become part of the virus? No other virus was known to do any such thing.

"Why does it produce this secreted glycoprotein in large

amounts?" asked Sanchez. "You can detect it in the blood of people infected. What is it doing? Does it have a role in the persistence of the virus in the natural host? In man, does it go out and bind to specific cells and turn them off? Does it intervene somehow?

"We don't know," he said. "We find that we're at the very beginning of understanding how these viruses operate."

There was one clue, however. When Sanchez and his colleagues compared the glycoprotein's genetic code with others on file in GenBank, a mammoth database of nucleic acid sequences, they found that the code contained a small region that was very similar to those of certain oncogenic retroviruses. Those retrovirus sequences had been shown to possess immunosuppressive properties: they weakened the action of the body's immune system, often with fatal results for the person involved. In the case of Ebola infections of humans, that same bit of extra genetic code might play a similar role, producing similar lethal effects. The secreted glycoproteins, in other words, might function as molecular shock troops, advance guards of chemical agents that went out and softened up the cells for invasion.

Maybe. No one really knew, and this, too, remained in the "unknown" category. As Sanchez's boss, C. J. Peters, once put it, "We're trying to figure out how these molecules affect the response of the infected human, but we haven't come up with anything except about five years' worth of experiments."

The apparent emergence of new diseases, illusory though it typically was, nevertheless seemed to require an "explanation." Why were all these strange "new" diseases showing up just now?

A popular answer was that by venturing out into nature's pastoral realms, we'd brought those diseases upon ourselves. Supposedly, our exposure to these deadly agents, and our suffering the diseases they caused, was nature's payback for our environmental crimes: we'd invaded the rain forests, mowed them down, and converted them into parking lots, strip malls, and endless McDonald's. If in the process we'd run up against a spate of new organisms that weren't especially agreeable to the human metabolism, well, why should we be in the least surprised?

Tempting as that reasoning might have been in the abstract, it didn't quite cover all cases: the Four Corners outbreak, for example, could not be made to fit the paradigm. For one thing, the initially affected population, the Navajo, was a race that had been in the area long before white Europeans ever set foot on the continent. The Navajo, furthermore, prided themselves upon living in harmony with nature. They worshiped nature, they regarded it as sacred, they venerated it. They did not rape, pillage, or otherwise violate the land.

The Navajo Reservation, moreover, was one of the least-developed areas of the American Southwest: there were no high-rise buildings, international airports, Jack Nicklaus golf courses, or Coca-Cola bottling plants anywhere within it. The reservation was crisscrossed by narrow and rutted dirt roads, and people got around in pickup trucks, four-wheel-drive vehicles, and sometimes even on horseback. Most of them lived simply in basic frame houses, mobile homes, or in hogans—small, earth-covered huts—in a sparsely populated red desert. The trailer that Merrill Bahe lived in was set well back from the road near the town of Little Water, total population 659.

Whatever else it was, the Four Corners outbreak was not a case of human beings invading nature and disturbing its kindly, retiring, and law-abiding pathogens. In fact, just the opposite was true: it was a case of nature's creatures invading long-established human homes.

As the Navajo tribal elders told the CDC investigators, heavy precipitation during the winter of 1993 produced a glut of piñon nuts, the main food of deer mice. Deer mice, as the CDC had learned, were the principal carriers of hantavirus. After the mouse population grew in response to the food surplus, the animals entered Navajo homes in great numbers. The mice shed the virus in their urine and droppings, and the Indians, unawares, started breathing the virus particles into their lungs. This was true in the Four Corners cases and it was true of the case in North Dakota.

So, try as you might, you couldn't blame those hantavirus deaths on the environmental callousness of human beings. The virus invaded people's homes, entered their bodies, and killed them.

11 The Grand Departure

When Joanna Buffington left work for the day, her practice was to walk out through the offices of the Special Pathogens Branch in the basement of Building 3. This was where C. J. Peters and Ali Khan were located, but that wasn't why she went out that way; rather, her bicycle was locked to the bike rack out there, and this was just the easiest route to take.

So on her way out she'd sail down the hallway past the hand-lettered sign that said THE HOT ZONE, Peters's punning memento of his role in the Reston affair (it also referred, one supposed, to the fever pitch of work being done in his offices), and she'd wave and say hi to Ali Khan, whom she'd known from her first days at CDC when both of them were still in EIS training.

At the beginning of the Kikwit outbreak, the basement of Building 3 was even more than the usual beehive: chirping telephones, people running from office to office, strangers roving through the hallways with Minicams and microphones, et cetera. Ali Khan, Joanna soon learned, was about to leave for Kikwit himself, a prospect that held no interest for her.

"I had absolutely no desire to go near that place," she recalled later. "Having just seen the movie *Outbreak* and read the books and knowing something about the 1976 Ebola epidemics from teaching the case studies, I thought, *I don't want to be near there at all.*"

Nevertheless, just as a joke she'd call out to Ali on her way past his office, *"Je parle français,* you know!" and Ali would reply, "Look, do you want to go? If you do, you're there. Just say the word." And Joanna would always answer, "No way!"

After all, it wasn't as if they needed her to go to Zaire: Ali and C. J. were swamped with requests. Besides, she had the July EIS course to teach, meaning that she couldn't leave now even if she wanted to.

But during the summer as more and more of her friends and colleagues went over to Kikwit and came back in one piece, she somewhat wistfully started thinking to herself, *Gee, you know, I missed this.* "And then I started thinking, *Well, what's my schedule like? I do all this work preparing for the summer course, I put the course on in July, and then . . . then in August I've got nothing to do.*"

Whereupon she decided that if anything was still going on in Kikwit during August, then she really ought to try to get herself shipped out to Africa.

"There'll be malaria and typhoid and probably a little Ebola around," she reasoned, "but that's not what I came to public health for, to be afraid of that stuff. I came to help respond to acute public health emergencies, whereas the last two years I've been in the office. I need to get out, I need to get back into the field again."

Which is how it transpired that on August 1, 1995, Joanna Buffington stepped off the Air Kasai DC-3 and first set foot on planet Kikwit.

Her assignment there, basically, was to close up shop. The CDC had been in the city continuously since May 12, other interested parties from all over the Western world had been overrunning the place since then, and by now the Zairians had had quite enough of all the attention. The last Ebola case had been identified, the patient had gone home cured, and the government wanted to declare the thing over and done with. In fact, the Zairians and the World Health Organization had settled on August 24 as the date upon which the epidemic would be pronounced dead, an occasion to be marked by grand celebrations and festivities, after which everyone would please go back to where they had come from, thanks just the same for all the help.

Still, the CDC had planned to be in the area well into the fall, doing animal and insect trapping, finishing up missing-link studies, occupational studies, risk-factor studies, cartographic studies, all sorts of other studies, plus serosurveys and whatever else, and suddenly all of it had to be compressed down into the space of a mere three weeks. Joanna Buffington, known far and wide for her tremendous organizational skills, would supervise the pullout operation and act as the overall deadline enforcer.

All the remaining CDC people, she decided, would depart from Kikwit the day after the celebration—there was just no reason to stay on after that. But that in turn meant that all the multifarious studies in progress would have to be concluded by then, no matter what. Above all, there could be nothing new: no new programs, surveys, tests, experiments, initiatives, or anything else that hadn't already been under way by the time she arrived. Nothing extra could be tacked on at the last moment. She'd hashed this out with her good friend Ali Khan and everybody else before she left Atlanta, and all of them agreed that this was to be the official policy.

What a surprise, then, that when Ali Khan rolled into Kikwit on August 14 for his second tour of duty, he produced out of his pocket a little white card listing a whole catalog of timely new research projects. He wanted to take bone marrow samples from the Ebola survivors, he wanted to expand the sero-surveys into a few of the outlying villages, so on and so forth.

Joanna Buffington listened to this enumeration of hopes and couldn't believe her ears. Supposedly, Ali was coming back just to help close things out, tidy up some loose ends, do this, that, and the other.

She said, "No! Absolutely not! Forget it! Nothing new, that was the agreement. The twenty-fifth of August, we're out of here."

"Please, I just want to do these few tiny little things," he said. "Just this and this and this and this. Come on, this stuff is really important."

"All right, fine," she said. "As long as we leave on the twenty-fifth. The twenty-fifth of August and we're out of here."

Ali's bone marrow project did not go well. The theory behind it was entirely sensible: the bone marrow contained the cells that had produced the antibodies that had saved the convalescents, the Ebola survivors, of whom there were now about seventy. Those antibodies, which had neutralized the Ebola virus particles circulating in their bloodstream, could also save the lives of future Ebola patients, if any. You'd simply harvest the antibodies from the bone marrow of the survivors, purify them, maybe engineer them a little, then inject them into the new victims, and they, too, perhaps, would be cured of the disease.

Ali had arranged for a physician to be flown in from Kinshasa, a hematologist by the name of Dr. Izzia, who would do the actual "aspirations," as they were called. He'd lay the patient down on a table, drape the person's body, scrub the chest area, and under local anesthetic he'd stick a hypodermic needle into the sternum and pull back on the plunger, withdrawing with it some of the bone marrow. Dr. Izzia, who was extremely experienced at this, was standing by even now, ready and waiting to do the procedure and then fly back to Kinshasa.

The patients, though, to put it mildly, were not especially receptive to the scheme. They were, after all, convalescents, which was to say that every last one of them had been ill with Ebola hemorrhagic fever, an experience memorable for its extreme unpleasantness. They'd all recovered from it in the past several weeks, and although they were now healthy again, indeed they were looking quite well, they were not particularly eager to hand themselves over to this new batch of white-coated Ebola docs, even if only for twenty minutes or so.

All of which was entirely understandable.

Ali Khan, nevertheless, attempted various heartfelt appeals.

"Look, the purpose of this is to benefit additional Zairians, additional Africans who may get the disease," he said. "I mean, this isn't going to benefit some Americans. This is going to benefit additional Zairians if we can find some sort of immune therapy to help patients."

But the answer was no.

Efficient as she was at finally getting people out of there on schedule, Joanna Buffington was near her wit's end just about the whole time she was in Kikwit. The place was plain hard on the nerves. This was true right from the beginning, starting with her very first night in the city, which she spent at the glorious and magnificent Hôtel Kwilu.

"Big mistake," she later confided. "The Inter-Continental was just outrageously overpriced but fairly comfortable. The Kwilu, I got a room on the second floor, facing the street. First big mistake."

People were out there on the street the whole night talking and arguing and shuffling around. There were shouts, whoops, trucks going by, diesel fumes, loud music, children crying, goats baaing, roosters crowing, chickens squawking.

The mosquito netting she'd put up in her room, meanwhile, kept falling down on her head, plus she worried about the

Kwilu's famous rat population and their habit of paying you regular nighttime visits. Cathy Merriman, she knew, had trapped a rat in her very own room while staying at the legendary Hôtel Kwilu.

Merriman was a Canadian bat biologist who'd come in with the ecological team to do bat-trapping work. She'd taken up residence at the Kwilu, where for two nights in a row at exactly three-thirty in the morning, she heard the sound of tiny rodent feet scraping their way up the wall behind the closet. Afterward, she found pieces of fruit lying nearby—bits of pineapple, banana, or whatever. The animal was clearly getting the fruit from someplace else (Merriman never kept any food in her room) and taking it back to the rat nest to snack on.

Merriman had always thought bats were incredibly neat, but she didn't much care for rats at all, and besides they were keeping her awake at night, so the next day she went over to George's house, where most of the CDC people were staying, and got an animal trap, a Sherman live-animal trap, from one of the rodent trappers. That night she baited it with some peanut butter, set it next to the closet, and went to sleep. Exactly three-thirty in the morning—*bang!*—the trap snapped shut, and milling around inside it was the catch of the day, an eight-inch-long brown rat. Merriman put the cage out in the hallway so she could sleep in peace for the rest of the night, and the next day she brought it over to the rodent trappers, who added the beast to their specimen collection.

Nor was she the only member of the animal team to have such wee-hours adventures at the Hôtel Kwilu. Andy Comer, a CDC entomologist, had also been hassled by visiting rodents. "Cathy caught hers on the first try," he admitted. "It took me several nights."

Joanna Buffington, luckily, never saw any rats during her stay at the Kwilu. Still, "I didn't sleep a wink that first night."

She later transferred out over to George's house, which had no rats, and which was further improved by a staff of twenty-four-hour-a-day security guards—"sentinels," armed soldiers—stationed outside the house to safeguard you against intruders or whatever. They constituted their own type of threat and muttered in low tones the entire night, but at least Joanna could sleep through that.

Wherever you were in Kikwit, though, getting the simplest things done was always a big problem.

"It is extraordinarily difficult to get things done in Kikwit," said a CDC physician who spent three weeks in the city. "I would often spend over an hour trying to print a document. One of the items discussed at length by the technical committee was how to assure that a committee member was not using AA flashlight batteries for personal use. It was decided that he would have to turn in his used batteries in order to get new batteries. One could not make a plan and then expect it to work without a high level of continued oversight. Things do not work in Kikwit, that's why they have an Ebola epidemic."

Getting a copying machine, fax machine, or satellite phone fixed in Kikwit was next to impossible, whereas all those things broke down with dependable regularity. Buying gasoline on Sunday was feasible *en principe*, as they said in Zaire, but nevertheless it required official permission slips and signatures and the payment of exorbitant "fees." Conversely, once certain procedures were actually under way, it took a miracle to get them stopped again. Some of the hired help, for example, couldn't be unhired, no matter what you told them: they'd just show up again for work the next day. Events in Kikwit tended to happen or terminate of their own inherent logic and momentum, they progressed impervious to direct human influence or control.

The general poverty was also a problem for many who spent time in the city, not excluding Joanna Buffington. She was a zealous environmentalist at home and considered herself an extremely conscientious recycler: she'd return plastic take-out containers to the local deli just so that the deli could use them again, but that was nothing compared to Kikwit.

"If you throw anything out that's not destroyed somehow— mechanically destroyed or burned—people will use it," she said. "The kids would reuse an ordinary plastic bag. They'd crumple it up and bind it with rubber bands and they'd use it as a soccer ball until it disintegrated. Any container that we emptied out would disappear, because everything had a use. The animal team would store animal samples and really nasty toxic chemicals in plastic bottles, and when they left, they said make sure you destroy them because otherwise people will use them for carrying water.

"I thought, *Well, that's kind of a shame,*" she added. "But we had to burn them or put holes in them so nobody could carry water in those bottles."

Harvesting antibodies from the bone marrow of Ebola survivors and injecting them into new patients was one possible means of curing them of the disease. In early June, Tamfum Muyembe had tried out a different, slightly riskier approach, taking whole blood from survivors and transfusing it into new patients. The hope was that they'd be cured by the same antibodies that had saved the survivors.

Essentially the same procedure had already been used in the case of Lassa fever when Jordi Casals, the Yale virologist, had contracted the disease in the lab. He'd been injected with some of Penny Pinneo's blood plasma, and he'd survived, just as she had. It had also been tried in the case of Ebola, when Geoffrey Platt accidentally injected himself with the virus at Porton Down and then fell ill with Ebola fever. He'd received transfusions of blood serum from patients who had recovered from the illness in Africa, and he, too, had survived the disease. A simple blood transfusion, then, might cure Ebola fever, and even if it didn't, it was in any case worth a try.

That was on the one hand. On the other hand, none of this had ever been tested scientifically on human patients: there'd been no control groups, the patients in question might have recovered on their own, and so on. And when the identical procedure had been tried on experimentally infected animal subjects, the animals died at the same rate as those that had not received the plasma, meaning that, as C. J. Peters expressed it, "all experimental animal data suggests that these modalities would have no effect."

Medically speaking, therefore, the blood-transfusion idea was roughly equivalent to an item of folklore, and when word finally reached WHO in Geneva that Muyembe was trying this out on some of his patients, there was a flurry of protest from headquarters.

So in June, Dr. Giorgio Torrigani, director of WHO's communicable diseases division, sent a fax to Muyembe in Kikwit laying out his concerns, saying that "we have no reason to believe that such treatment will be effective." To begin with, he said, the procedure had not been effective in animal tests, but even if it *had* been effective, the scheme still had potential risks. For one thing, the doctors in Kikwit could not be absolutely sure that a suspected Ebola patient was actually suffering from Ebola as opposed to shigella, yellow fever, or whatever. Only blood tests could confirm the diagnosis, and these still had to be performed in well-equipped laboratories such as those at the CDC. To transfuse a patient who was only *suspected* of Ebola, then, was to treat a patient who might not in fact have the disease in the first place. That, in turn, was highly risky because the donor's blood might contain not only antibodies to Ebola, but also the Ebola virus itself, meaning that you might end up giving the disease to a patient who did not originally have it.

Beyond that, the donor's blood might harbor other noxious viruses, hepatitis B, for example, or even HIV, which caused AIDS. It was entirely possible that you'd not only fail to cure the patient of Ebola, but that you'd give him either hepatitis or AIDS or both. WHO was willing to provide Muyembe with test kits that would screen the donors' blood for hepatitis B and HIV, said Torrigani, "but providing these kits is in no way meant to indicate that we believe the procedure will have any benefit."

All those considerations notwithstanding, Muyembe and the other Zairian doctors decided to take the gamble, and on June 6, 1995, a patient named Nicole Nganga, a twenty-seven-year-old woman, was transfused with blood taken from a thirty-three-year-old male survivor by the name of Emery Nikolo. Nikolo had fallen ill with Ebola on April 28, recuperated, and was then out of danger. Nicole Nganga first manifested hemorrhagic fever symptoms on May 30, which meant that by the time she was transfused with four hundred milliliters of Nikolo's blood, she was more than a week into the illness. But she survived the transfusion and completely recovered from Ebola fever.

The Zairian doctors ended up transfusing a total of eight patients with blood taken from Ebola survivors, and seven out of the eight lived, which translated out to a mortality rate of only 12.5 percent as compared to a rate of 77 percent for untreated patients. To all appearances, then, this was indeed some sort of a cure. Further, when blood samples from all those eight patients were finally tested back at the CDC, all eight samples were found to be positive for Ebola, which meant that in no case was Muyembe treating patients who hadn't really been suffering from the disease.

Still, there were other possible explanations for this seemingly miraculous recovery rate.

"Some of them were apparently treated while getting better," said Ali Khan—meaning that they might have recovered on their own, without the blood transfusions.

"In addition," he said, "if the therapy was successful, it may have been due to the concurrently transfused leukocytes [white blood cells]"—instead of due to Ebola-virus antibodies.

But none of this altered the final numbers. The fact was that in the middle of the Kikwit Ebola crisis, seven out of the eight patients who'd been transfused with convalescent blood ultimately walked out of Kikwit General Hospital under their own power—an otherwise exceedingly rare event.

Friday, August 18, was Joanna Buffington's birthday: she was thirty-seven years old. Everybody was so busy working that day, however, that a celebration was postponed till the very end of the week, Sunday. Ali Khan had the idea of giving her as a present Kikwit's renowned boat-ride excursion, an evening water-taxi ride on the river Kwilu, the waterway after which the fabulous Hôtel Kwilu had been named. A fleet of dugout canoes, also known as pirogues, went out on the river where they were pushed along by poles wielded by these allegedly expert river boatmen, who at one point were supposed to start caroling the passengers with a variety of traditional African songs.

Well, it sounded wonderful. It would be like a Venetian gondola cruise, only on the river Kwilu—just incredibly pretty, a peaceful sunset float through the jungle.

And so on Sunday afternoon, toward dusk, everybody drove over to the river: Ali and Joanna, who were the only two CDC people left in Kikwit; Ali's interpreter, Mahuma; Yon Fleerackers, from the Institute of Tropical Medicine in Antwerp; plus a few other hardworking and longtime members of the Ebola team.

Before they even reached the river, though, some subtle signs indicated that this, too, would be another classic Kikwit fiasco.

"We were late getting started," Joanna remembered. "It's late afternoon Sunday, these clouds were coming in, black clouds, it's getting dark, and there's thunder and lightning, and I'm thinking, *This is stupid, we should not be going out on the water."*

No one else, apparently, shared those feelings. "It's your birthday!" Ali Khan kept saying.

Supposedly, the boat was just down the hill: you parked the car, walked down the bank, and hopped in the canoe. In actual fact the boat landing was a mile and a half away, which meant a long trek through the woods, through fields that were being burned for cultivation. The sky was already a deep pink, the sun was setting behind the pall of smoke, they were following this dim little path through the burning landscape, Ali in sneakers, Joanna in sandals, fire and fumes on both sides, gusts of wind coming up, rumbles of low thunder off in the distance, and . . .

This is really stupid, Joanna Buffington thought to herself.

But they made it to the boat and clambered in. And then, just after they'd pushed off from the shore, the sky opened up. It was the normal African rainfall, the usual submersion, as if the clouds had exploded directly overhead, but all of it was now magnified out of proportion by the fact of being out on the water in the dark, drifting around on a forgotten jungle river in the middle of nowhere.

"The winds are whipping up and I'm saying, *This is the end of my life.* My life is flashing before my eyes, and I think, *No one will ever feel sorry for me if they look at all these risk factors."*

Within minutes the boat's got a pool of water sloshing around in the bottom and everybody's drenched to the skin. The expert boatmen pay no attention. Outside the boat, little wavelets of brown, muddy river water are splashing up and coming in over the side, Joanna's sitting there in the bow shivering, she's absolutely freezing by this point, gripping the edge with her white-knuckled hands, she's thinking, *We're all going to die!* when somebody calls out, *"Look in the water! A hippopotamus!"*

A hippopotamus!

Somebody screams.

And suddenly this huge black shape was coming right at them, bobbing up and down in the river, ripples of black water spilling off its back, it *bumps* against the boat, and . . .

Joanna thinks, *Now we are definitely going to die.*

Insofar as the official formalities went, the epidemic would be over when a period of twice the virus's maximum incubation period had elapsed from the date of the last known case without any new cases being reported in the interim. The Ebola virus's maximum incubation period was twenty-one days, which meant that forty-two days after the death (or recovery) of the last case, the epidemic would be over, finally, once and for all.

The last known case of Ebola hemorrhagic fever in Kikwit was a twenty-two-year-old unmarried male by the name of Marcel Mupalanga Masemo. Masemo had been admitted to Kikwit General Hospital on June 24 with a temperature of 103° F, vertigo, muscle aches, weakness, and other assorted signs and symptoms, but neither hemorrhaging nor diarrhea. These did not necessarily add up to Ebola—he was even given quinine, as if he had malaria—but the epidemiological clues were more clear-cut. During the first part of June, Masemo had been taking care of his cousin Trégine, a nine-year-old girl who had died of Ebola fever on June 11. He'd helped her feed herself and get up and move around and had several times been in direct contact with the stomach contents she'd vomited up.

He'd been placed in Pavilion 3, the Ebola ward, and over the next three weeks he'd gotten steadily better, his signs and symptoms slowly disappearing until, on Friday, July 14, he was removed from Pavilion 3 and transferred to the convalescent ward, where he'd recuperated on his own.

On July 15, Pavilion 3 was empty of patients. Later, it and

217

Pavilion 2, which had also housed Ebola victims, were officially closed and then both were clinically disinfected. The countdown to Ebola-free status, meanwhile, had begun on July 14 and would end on August 24, the forty-second day thereafter, with a big celebration, a *grande fête*.

August 22 was a Day of Remembering in Kikwit. In commemoration of the Ebola victims, music and dance were prohibited in the city. The next day, a Wednesday, families placed flowers on the graves of those who had died. And then it was August 24, a Thursday, the Day of Proclamation of Ebola-Free Status, day of the *grande fête*.

Dawn broke gray and overcast, with a dull, milky white glare that was slightly painful on the eyes. The airport was packed by eight in the morning, the locals having arrived by foot, on bicycles, in cars, in the backs of pickup trucks, even in dump trucks, to welcome Zaire's public health officialdom. The place was chock-full of Kikwitians, all of them now waiting for the special charter flight of the Air Kasai DC-3, the one that was bringing in Tamfum Muyembe; Dr. Ebrahim Samba, the WHO regional director for Africa; Lynette Simon of the USAID; ambassadors from Belgium, France, Italy, and a few African states, plus sundry other government dignitaries, all of them coming to Kikwit to celebrate the final victory over the virus.

There were banners, flags, music, and folk dancers. A military drill team was on the field marching around and doing formations.

The plane arrived, there were mass greetings, and then the health worthies were driven over to Kikwit General Hospital. Here there was a Procession of the Ebola-Fighters, a public display in which the entire hospital staff was decked out in full viral battle array: gowns, aprons, gloves, helmets, face masks. They were lined up in front of Pavilion 10, the *salle d'urgence*, color by color, the Red Cross in bright orange jumpsuits and black rubber boots, the nurses in yellow gowns and white plastic caps, others in spiffy blue jackets and white pants. From the looks of them, these people were ready for anything.

On the ground front and center was a red stretcher with what appeared to be a black body bag laid out on top of it; standing next to it was a gowned attendant with a sprayer unit on his back, the omnipresent bleach-sprayer. The bleach-sprayer was the single most lasting symbol of everything that had gone on at Kikwit General: he was the cleansing force, the agent of purity, the virus killer.

The party of bigwigs then moved off to the actual proclamation site, which of course was the fabled and magical Hôtel Kwilu. They made speeches. They signed the official document, the "Declaration of the End of Ebola Hemorrhagic Fever in Kikwit." And they handed out certificates to the various Ebola-fighters.

Ali Khan and Joanna Buffington, when their names were called, were not among those present.

Then there was lunch.

Later, at the soccer field, there was a Tournoi Ebola—an Ebola Tournament—once more commemorating the final victory over the virus. Later still there was supposed to be a march through town, a sort of spontaneous street demonstration of thanksgiving for deliverance from Ebola. The street demonstration, though, never materialized.

And then it was August 25, departure day for Ali and Joanna.

For them, everything had worked out well enough. Ali finally got his bone-marrow samples. After they'd initially refused to cooperate, the convalescents had gone home for the night and had apparently rethought the matter. Anyway, four of them were back the next morning, and they now agreed to the procedure, giving Ali the specimens he wanted.

Even Joanna's birthday celebration on the river Kwilu had worked out for the best: the "hippopotamus" had actually been an overturned pirogue that had just been bumping along in the water. The storm moved off, the skies cleared, the stars came out, and the expert boatmen began singing. Truly, it had been an incredible evening.

They'd missed the awards ceremony at the Hôtel Kwilu, but only because they'd been working like crazy to clear out of Kikwit. They were running around packing, collecting supplies, files, samples, working right up till the last minute. By the time they got to the banquet room, the hotel had run out of food.

Of course, this being Kikwit, a couple of things had not worked out exactly as planned. The "last case," for one thing, had not been the last case. Another case cropped up about a week after Marcel Masemo's, and—worst of all—nobody recognized it for what it was: Ebola.

"That was unfortunate, that there was a case in Kikwit but it didn't ring any bells among people," Ali Khan said later. "There was a woman who was pregnant and she'd died with really good-sounding symptoms for Ebola hemorrhagic fever— she'd actually been *in contact* with somebody with Ebola hemorrhagic fever—but no bells went off in anybody's head, nobody said, 'Oh, my God, this woman may have Ebola hemorrhagic fever!' It's unfortunate that in a town that's as sensitized as this one, nobody realized that this was the real thing. That was kind of discouraging."

And then there'd been the morning-of-departure mix-up. It had actually begun the day before, when George, the owner of George's house, presented Joanna with a last-minute bill.

"It was a bill for repairing the freezer," Joanna said. "It was for several thousand zaires, which translated into a couple of hundred dollars. And we get this bill and I said, '*Freezer?* We don't even *have* a freezer! This lousy refrigerator's only on for a couple of hours a day, we don't even have the power you're supposed to be supplying us with from the generator. What is this about a *freezer?*' "

The story was that there actually *had* been a freezer, the CDC people were storing their samples in it, but then one day it had stopped working. George said he'd repair it but it was going to cost a lot, and anyway nobody ever saw the freezer again. End of the freezer bill.

But then there'd been the *water* bill, which a man from the Kikwit water-supply company, such as it was, presented to Joanna the day before departure.

"This water bill was predicted to be maybe two hundred dollars, which is a lot," Joanna said. "I mean they're already socking us—two hundred dollars is the annual per capita income in Zaire. But we get a water bill for seven hundred and sixty-three dollars and I said, no way. This is ridiculous. And the rate, it said, 'Commercial rate, fifty thousand zaires per unit,' as opposed to the residential rate, which is something like three and a half thousand. So, three point five thousand up to fifty thousand per unit. And I said this is complete abuse. And I said we are not going to pay this, we are not commercial."

Next morning, their final day in the city, the day Ali and Joanna are leaving the place once and for all, the guy from the water commission rides up on his motorbike, he comes to George's house to collect his money, for water billed at the commercial rate.

"But we're not commercial!" Joanna says.

"But this is commercially *zoned,*" the man says.

"Look, we're here in humanitarian response to a medical emergency, and this is a *household.*"

"Well, it's commercially zoned. How do I know you're not selling things from the house?"

Selling things from the house?

Joanna drove over to see the commandant himself, Mayor Mavita, over at the Hôtel de Ville.

"Oh, don't worry," said Mayor Mavita. "I'll take care of this."

Still, Joanna left the money with someone else, she left the whole amount at the commercial rate, just in case the CDC was legally responsible for the water bill . . . in case they'd been *selling things from the house.*

And that was their grand departure.

12 The Golden Age of Virus Paranoia

par•a•noi•a *n.* A nondegenerative, limited, usually chronic psychosis characterized by delusions of persecution or of grandeur, strenuously defended by the afflicted with apparent logic and reason.
—*The American Heritage Dictionary.* 2nd College Edition. 1982.

In 1996, the CDC got its latest and grandest facility, a new administration building. Six stories of glass and concrete, it was the newest structure to rise on the campus since the Viral and Rickettsial Diseases Laboratory, Building 15, opened for business in 1988.

The surprise was that this new structure was actually numbered Building 16, the next in numerical sequence. One thing there was no obvious logic to at the Centers for Disease Control was building numerology, and at one point in the late 1970s, no one could remember exactly when or at whose order, some of the building numbers were changed. Building 5 (the Virus Disease Building) suddenly became Building 7; Building 6 (the Power Plant) became Building 11; and so on. Some numbers were skipped, and there were no buildings numbered 12 or 13 on the Clifton Road grounds. As to *why* the numbers were changed, what the theoretical *purpose* of it was . . .

"I have no idea," said David Sencer, former director of the CDC. "*No* idea. I'm sure there was some rhyme or reason for it, I don't know what it was."

ED REGIS

Whatever the rhyme or reason, the effect of it was to cause confusion ever afterward, at least for those who'd lived through the changeover, which decidedly took some getting used to. John Richardson, the retired director of laboratory safety, was playing poker one night with some old friends of his from the CDC; they were trying to recall how the new numbering scheme differed from the old one, and they got exactly nowhere. "For one thing, we were playing poker," he said. "Besides, it wasn't all that important, nothing hinged on it. Still, we couldn't remember the numbers."

"People have to tell me what a given building is by describing it," said Dave Sencer. "I don't know the numbering system."

Impenetrable as it was, this was just one more essentially harmless example of modern bureaucracy at work, and other than for the befuddlement it occasioned on the part of staff, visitors, and historians of the place, it made no real difference to anything. Another bureaucratic artifact, however, had more serious repercussions on the way things went, and this was the CDC's relentless mission creep, its internecine growth, its tendency to keep taking on new responsibilities right and left, no matter what. The CDC was a place that just never said no: miscellaneous programs, institutes, initiatives, centers, functions, projects, offices, departments, sections, commissions, activities, branches, services, and whatever else gravitated toward Atlanta like the big Delta passenger jets that flew into Hartsfield hour by hour. They just kept coming on in, one after another, bingo, and they were incorporated into the huge, growing ectoplasm like germs gobbled up by a macrophage. The CDC was an octopus, and in classic bureaucratic fashion, it *grew*.

By 1994, the agency that had started out in life as a simple and narrow-purpose malaria-eradication agency had enlarged, expanded, and amplified itself into an organization with seven separate "centers." At that point, the "centers" of the Centers for Disease Control and Prevention were: the National Center for Chronic Disease Prevention and Health Promotion, the National Center for Environmental Health, the National Center for Health Statistics, the National Center for Infectious Diseases, the National Center for Injury Prevention and Control, the National Center for Prevention Services, and the National Institute for Occupational Safety and Health.

And those were only the "centers." There was more to the CDC than that: there was the Epidemiology Program Office, the International Health Program Office, the Public Health Practice Program Office, and the National Immunization Program. There was also the Agency for Toxic Substances and Disease Registry, and each and every one of these various centers, institutes, offices, and registries had its own long list of sub-offices, divisions, programs, et cetera.

One could not say of the CDC, however, that the place had "lost direction." To the contrary, it *took on* directions, it added them, it went off in all directions, it went everywhere and tried to do everything, all at once. It embraced every new function in sight, no matter how foreign to its original purpose or how tenuous its relation to public health—family planning, for example—or to the people whose health it was designed to protect, which was to say, Americans. The CDC went all over the globe, conducting health workshops, training programs, management assistance courses in Latin America, Africa, and Asia. It sponsored "worksite lifestyle programs" and had a separate project for "preventing homicide in the workplace." It implemented "a ten-month fellowship in health and religion for a minister from the Congress of the National Black Church." (Health and *religion?*) It funded "an ethnographic study of Hispanic/Latino men in southeastern Texas and southern California who do not identify themselves as gay but who have sex with other men."

This major diffusion of its mission and functions, if it had to be located in time, blossomed in 1978, with the CDC's Red

Book Committee, a group of sixteen outside experts hired by the incoming director, Bill Foege, as prelude to his "complete reorganization" of the place. This was the study group that had narrowly escaped listing hernia as a major national health problem; those problems that did make the final cut, however, brought some strange new animals into the public health arena: smoking, motor vehicle accidents, social disorders, and "stress." Later, Foege and some other CDC administrators added violence and unwanted pregnancy to the roster.

"Of all the areas, violence was the most controversial," said Elizabeth Etheridge, the CDC's official historian, "and the one that the public health community found hardest to accept."

And with good reason: whatever else could be said about it, violence was a product of human free choice, not something that was transmitted to you unknowingly or against your will, like a virus. You did not wake up in the morning and find yourself suddenly in the grip of a violence infection. One could of course speak *metaphorically*—you could speak of an "epidemic" of violence, of a community "plagued" by violence, and so on—but still and all, these were no more than figures of speech, and everyone knew that you could not literally catch a "violence disease." Violence, however, now became another item on CDC's progressively ever more crowded agenda.

The upshot of all this inclusion of extra functions and metaphorical new "plagues" was that by 1994 the CDC's main business, the control of infectious diseases, was just one of dozens of jobs that the CDC had taken on, just another of its many and diffuse assignments. At that point, indeed, the National Center for Infectious Diseases, the NCID, was receiving only about 10 percent of the CDC's overall budget. Ninety percent of the money that came into the CDC, in other words, went to other places than to the NCID.

One might well wonder, therefore, whether the CDC's historic role of controlling infectious diseases was being diluted, weakened, or undermined by the pull of its other assorted and copious tasks. The people who worked at the NCID would eventually complain that they were being "stretched thin," that they didn't have enough money, enough resources, enough manpower, to do their jobs properly. They were barely in control of the situation. They had no cushion beneath them, there was no backup, no personnel redundancy in the event of a crisis. The fact was that they had become just one more subspecialty in an already top-heavy bureaucratic structure.

As to whether this proliferation of purposes, mission, and institutional attention had any effect on the rate of infectious disease within the American population, the answer was not long in coming. In 1996, a group of CDC researchers published, in *The Journal of the American Medical Association (JAMA)*, an article entitled "Trends in infectious disease mortality in the United States." Six of the article's seven coauthors worked at the NCID, and one of them, Ruth Berkelman, was the NCID's deputy director. The group had reviewed mortality data from the years 1980 to 1992, a time span that corresponded to the CDC's having taken on major new obligations in the wake of the 1978 Red Book Committee report, and found that during that period, infectious diseases had actually been on the rise. "Despite historical predictions that infectious diseases would wane in the United States," they said, "these data show that infectious diseases mortality in the United States has been increasing in recent years."

Given the expansion of the CDC's activities from its original purpose of controlling infectious diseases in the United States, that result was not wholly surprising.

Deflected though it was from its exclusive focus on infectious diseases, the CDC nevertheless had been fairly successful in wiping out many of them from the United States, or at least in cutting them down toward the vanishing point. In fact, one reason why the CDC had felt justified in widening the scope of its interests to include other things was the magnitude of the public health community's achievements in keeping epidemic infectious diseases at bay. Malaria was virtually gone from the country. Polio was a thing of the past. Smallpox had been removed from the planet. Rabies deaths were highly unusual. Diphtheria, of which there had been an average of fifteen thousand annual cases during the World War II years, was by the time the 1990s rolled around a disease that many younger Americans had never even heard of, much less ever suffered from, and in 1993 not a single case of diphtheria had been reported anywhere in the country. Yellow fever had just about vanished. In 1963, before the advent of widespread measles vaccinations, there had been some half million annual cases of the disease in the United States; in 1994, there were 301 reported cases of measles. *Haemophilus influenzae*, the primary cause of bacterial meningitis and a contributing cause of other childhood diseases, had been virtually eliminated from the country.

Life-threatening epidemics, which throughout all past history were considered "normal," "natural," and inescapable facts of human existence, had largely passed from the scene, and the American public no longer lived in fear of them. Cholera epidemics were unknown. Bubonic plague, which had once wiped out a third of Europe, had been reduced to the point that forty cases in the United States was deemed an intolerably high number, this despite the fact that the disease was easily treatable and there were virtually no deaths.

In 1900, the three leading causes of death in the United States were tuberculosis, pneumonia, and diarrheal enteritis—all three of them infectious diseases. By 1992, the three leading causes of death were heart disease, cancer, and stroke—none of them infectious diseases. Infectious diseases, including AIDS, at that point caused only 5 percent of all deaths; one of the biggest national health problems in the 1990s, indeed, was obesity.

Further, the "new" infectious diseases—hantavirus, Legion-naires', and Lyme disease, for example—did not remotely begin to approach the "old" ones in terms of the numbers of people they killed. During the 1918 influenza crisis, half a million Americans had died; hantavirus, by contrast, was known to have affected a total of 133 people in the United States and to have killed 66, starting from the original Four Corners out-break in 1993.

Except for influenza and AIDS, the country no longer had *epidemics*, it had *outbreaks*. But even AIDS, the new scourge, was nothing like the major killers of past history.

"AIDS is what we principally have on our minds at the mo-ment," said disease historian William McNeill at Stephen Morse's landmark Emerging Viruses conference in 1989. "But I must say that it is a poor country cousin in terms of the slowness of its propagation and the obviousness of behavioral adjustments that would check its spread. . . . It is always worth reminding oneself that more people die of automobile acci-dents each year than—I think it is still correct to say—have yet died of AIDS in the United States. Demographically, in terms of its effect on population, it is not yet a major phenomenon."

Five years later, by 1994, total cumulative U.S. AIDS deaths were 270,533; in that same year, however, 32,330 people died of AIDS while 43,000 died in traffic accidents. Still, the spread of AIDS could be, and in fact had been, curtailed by "behav-ioral adjustments," and this was a disease in which human behavior, as much as the virus itself, played a major role.

As for the higher infectious disease mortality rates that the CDC group had reported in the *JAMA* study, the increase did not constitute a huge rise in terms of absolute numbers of people, although when expressed in terms of percentages the results admittedly sounded alarming, as for example: "The rate of death due to septicemia increased 83 percent."

That sounded bad, taken by itself: an 83 percent increase!

But what that percentage actually amounted to was an increase from 4.2 deaths per 100,000 population to 7.7 deaths per 100,000 population. In other words, in a city roughly the size of Springfield, Illinois, or Abilene, Texas, there were an additional 3.5 deaths due to septicemia (blood poisoning) per year. Unsatisfactory as that was, it did not connote quite the same apparent catastrophe as "an increase of 83 percent." That the actual numbers involved were as small as they were only served to highlight the strictness of the standards against which the public's health was being measured in the 1990s.

At the end of the century, the CDC was assisting in the World Health Organization's program to eradicate polio from the entire world by the year 2000, a project that was nearly on schedule and which would repeat the successful drive against smallpox. Beyond that, it was looking forward to eradicating dracunculiasis (guinea-worm infection) and measles. But as far as disease eradication was concerned, the CDC had no definite plans, and no immediate higher goals, after that, and the place as a whole seemed to have suffered a crisis of self-confidence in relation to the diseases it was sworn to combat. Its aspirations had fallen a long way from the heyday health utopianism of the 1960s when people had spoken of completely wiping out infectious diseases by the end of the century. In 1996, by contrast, the CDC's newest director, David Satcher, was quoted as saying: "We know we will never conquer infectious diseases. The question is whether we can control these organisms so we can coexist."

We will never conquer infectious diseases.

For the head of the nation's premier disease-fighting agency, it was an awfully strange statement.

When Joanna got home from Kikwit, she cried for a good while.

"The first weekend back, I was kind of a wreck," she said.

"It was sort of relief, an incredible relief that I *have* things, and that I can *waste* things, mixed with a feeling of guilt. We came to Kikwit, we addressed this acute problem they had over there, but there was a much bigger chronic problem that we couldn't do much about, and that was poverty. And so we left: we went back home to our electricity, our money, our McDonald's, and we left them with what they had before Ebola, which is nothing. And that was very stressful for me. It just reminds you so much of how lucky we are, and that we can be wasteful. I mean I couldn't wait to get out of there in some ways, but a piece of me is still there. It was pretty overwhelming."

On a personal level, what the CDC physicians, virologists, and ecological team members brought back with them from Kikwit were memories, pictures, and "Ebola dolls." But what they really went over there for, and what they brought back with them as working scientists, was information, data, and biological samples, the latter of which they'd carted away in large numbers. They came back with almost thirty thousand insects: 28,664 by actual count, of mosquitoes, ticks, bedbugs, sand flies, tsetse flies, lice, and fleas. They took away hundreds of small-animal samples, from rats, mice, bats, shrews, domestic animals, monkeys, birds, snakes, and lizards, plus a large collection of what might be called "miscellaneous" (and in some cases even unknown) animals. There were more than three thousand of those specimens, all told.

In addition to the insects and animals, the researchers brought back with them from Kikwit approximately seven thousand human specimens: blood samples, stool samples, vomit and urine samples, and swabs of assorted other secretions, along with Ali Khan's hard-won bone marrow aspirates. That made for a combined grand total of some forty thousand specimens of various types that they'd taken away from the city and the jungles around Kikwit and brought back with them to Atlanta.

The hope had been, of course, that the CDC's lab workers would find the Ebola virus lurking in one or more of those animal and insect samples, thereby discovering at long last the natural reservoir of the virus.

By mid-1996, however, absolutely no trace of the virus had shown up anywhere—more proof, if anyone needed it, that the Ebola virus, like its cousin Marburg, was an extremely marginal commodity in nature.

The major remaining question was: What did it all mean? What was the significance, if any, insofar as public health was concerned, of the 1995 Ebola outbreak in Kikwit? Some public health officials, at the beginning, had made some fairly rash pronouncements, especially those on the order of "This is the big one," which turned out to be just a wee bit of an overstatement. Even Bill Clinton had used some fateful terms when, in a June 26, 1995, speech commemorating the fiftieth birthday of the United Nations, he spoke of "fatal diseases like the Ebola virus that could have threatened an entire continent."

An entire continent? Well, maybe. But the truth was that these and other such apocalyptic claims were tokens of an emerging new paradigm concerning the fundamental meaning of disease as well as its ultimate cause, the microbes. Disease, according to this new view, was not merely an artifact of biodiversity, a by-product of our sharing the planet with lots of other life-forms including rickettsias, bacteria, and viruses. No. Disease was, instead, an independent power, a corrective force, a moralistic and vengeful influence. It was nature's way of defending itself against invasive and unsightly humans.

This was the viewpoint that had been expressed by Richard Preston in The Hot Zone: "In a sense, the earth is mounting an immune response against the human species," he'd said. "Perhaps the biosphere does not 'like' the idea of five billion humans. . . . The earth's immune system, so to speak, has recognized the presence of the human species and is starting to kick in. The earth is attempting to rid itself of an infection by the human parasite."

Not only was it attempting to do so, it was actually succeeding in the attempt, at least according to Laurie Garrett in *The Coming Plague:* "That humanity had grossly underestimated the microbes was no longer, as the world approached the twenty-first century, a matter of doubt," she said. "The microbes were winning." (How it could be that the microbes were "winning" when the average life expectancy of the world's population steadily increased, when childhood mortality rates steadily decreased, when the global population spiraled forever upward, and when Africa, home of the world's most lethal viruses, had the world's highest rate of population growth year after year, was a mystery. It was during the years of the Black Plague, when the world's population actually *declined,* that the microbes were "winning.")

So radical and sweeping was this new paradigm that it represented a revised conception of nature itself. Nature, not so very long ago, had been regularly portrayed as "fragile." This was the conventional wisdom, it was the orthodox, established, and canonical view. The ecosystem, supposedly, was in a condition of such delicate equipoise that the slightest perturbation could wreak havoc and ruin everything. That was why nature had to be conserved, saved, and protected, after all, because nature was so very "fragile."

Well, nature was fragile no longer. Somehow, it had rallied. It had rebounded, snapped back, and gathered together its strength, to the point that the same natural world that formerly had to be protected from humanity had suddenly become humankind's chief exterminator. Far from being fragile, nature was now almighty and vindictive. And it was highly intolerant of its very own creation, people.

As were the microbes themselves. All at once viruses had replaced the A-bomb as the object of the apocalyptic vision.

No more would doomsday appear in the form of ballistic missiles raining death from out of the clouds; instead, destruction would rise up out of the rain forests in an act of viral correction and punishment. "AIDS is the revenge of the rain forest," Preston had written. "It is only the first act of the revenge."

So when Ebola once again crawled out of the primeval jungle and started killing people in Kikwit, what could it be but the fulfillment of a prophecy, the final act in the unfolding drama? What could it mean but that The End was Nigh?

Who could blame the public, then, when an Internet discussion group was created under the title "The Ebola virus—the end of the civilized world?" and people began saying things like:

> That the Ebola virus is a terrible threat to mankind is undoubtable, but I wonder if anybody has thought about the consequences of an epidemic disaster in areas with high concentration of population—for example central Europe or the eastern coast of the USA.
>
> Ebola kills 88 percent of the victims, and thus would such a populated area be reduced to almost nothing. . . .
>
> Indeed, Ebola is the mightiest threat mankind has faced yet.

And so on.

The only trouble with all this foaming viral paranoia was that it had nothing to do with reality. It was, instead, the stuff of legend. It was Hollywood, it was the movies, it was box office.

Indeed it was worse than that. The "revenge of the rain forest" doctrine was in fact a return to a prescientific, animistic conception of nature: it was a throwback to the days when the gods were portrayed as stomping about in heaven and hurling thunderbolts down from the sky. The only difference was that these days they were slinging viruses.

The world's virologists themselves soon rose up against the oncoming tide of virus paranoia, and it was symbolically fitting that some of the most vocal among them were located in Africa, the very place where the fabled viruses hailed from. Margaretha Isaäcson, the South African physician who'd stopped the transmission of Ebola virus at Ngaliema Hospital in Kinshasa during the original 1976 outbreak, said:

> Ebola is of absolutely no danger to the world at large. It is a dangerous virus, but it's relatively rare and quite easily contained.
> The virus needs the right conditions to multiply, whatever the virus is, be it Ebola or plague. It's not enough to just have the accident. The virus must first find itself in a favorable environment before it can affect anyone. The media is scaring the world out of its wits, and movies like *Outbreak* are doing people a great disservice.

Ed Rybicki, a virologist at the University of Cape Town, said:

> The town of Kikwit has a population of five hundred thousand and extremely poor medical treatment centers, and yet only three hundred people died there. That is not anywhere near 90 percent of the entire population.
> A simple yet very obvious statement of the facts. So if 499,700 people in Kikwit DIDN'T get Ebola, why are Americans so worried????

Indeed. The fact of the matter was that Ebola hemorrhagic fever, along with Marburg and Lassa, were diseases of poverty and bad hospitals. Although they thrived momentarily when they erupted in such environments, those same viruses were stopped cold every time they turned up in well-equipped medical institutions, whether in developed countries or elsewhere. When Marburg, the first of the unholy trio, showed up in Germany in 1967, it infected one round of twenty-five people, seven of whom died, then spread to six secondary cases among medical personnel and family members, all of whom lived. And that was the end of the Marburg epidemic.

The original Marburg incident was, and would remain, the largest human outbreak of any African hemorrhagic fever ever to appear in the developed West, and the virus had killed just seven people. Both Lassa and Ebola, the two other African hemorrhagic fever viruses, would arrive in Europe and the United States on several later occasions, but in none of those instances was there more than a single death, and in no case was there person-to-person transmission of the virus. When in 1969 Penny Pinneo was brought to the Columbia Presbyterian Medical Center New York with Lassa fever, there were no cases of secondary transmission. In 1976, when Geoffrey Platt contracted Ebola in a London lab, the infection started and ended with him. When Lassa was brought into a suburban Chicago hospital in 1989, it got no farther than the first case. And in 1994 when a Swiss primate researcher with Ebola hemorrhagic fever was admitted to the University Hospital of Basel, the patient recovered and the infection stopped then and there.

All of which suggested that these African hemorrhagic fever viruses were something less than omnipotent agents hell-bent on wiping out humankind. They were, in fact, dead chemicals. They were physical entities, particles of matter that, clever as they were on the molecular level and whatever neat tricks of information coding they were capable of, still had to obey all the normal laws of chemistry and physics. They still had to get from one person to the next before they could do further damage, and they could be prevented from doing so by the placement of simple physical barriers between them. Common and ordinary items such as rubber gloves, plastic gowns, and face masks could halt an epidemic. A killer virus could itself be killed by a liberal application of household bleach. Precisely those items, mundane and boring as they were, had been the very things that had terminated the Ebola outbreak in Kikwit.

Bernard Le Guenno, after he got back to Paris from Zaire, was invited to speak to scientific groups to tell about his findings and experiences in Kikwit. When he gave his talks, he'd illustrate his comments with a slide show, with pictures of the hospital and the city, plus charts and graphs showing the epidemic curve of the outbreak, the various lines of transmission, and so on. He'd project these images up on the screen to reinforce the different points he wanted to make.

Toward the very end of his talk he showed a slide on which appeared, in French, the single question: "Ebola virus infection—a menace to humanity?"

The next slide in sequence showed only one word: *"Non!"*

Epilogue: Submerging Diseases

The idea that a given virus might become extinct, not through intentional disease-eradication attempts, but just by itself, naturally and normally and in the ordinary course of events, was not often entertained during the golden age of virus paranoia, when "new" viruses were seen lurking under every stone. But the prospect of virus extinction was entirely genuine: it was an outgrowth of evolution by natural selection, a corollary of the fact that species evolved from other forms of life, enjoyed their brief heyday periods, then passed out of existence. Indeed, it was a commonplace observation among evolutionary biologists that many more species had evolved and become extinct than existed at any one time, including the present, and it was an accepted piece of conventional wisdom that species were becoming extinct at an ever more rapid pace, particularly those that lived in the rain forests.

Why, then, shouldn't those same extinctions include viruses?

"I'm sure it's got to be the case," said Rockefeller University virologist Stephen Morse. "But of course extinctions of pathogens are hard to document: they are noted only as apparent disappearance, and we cannot easily distinguish actual extinction from 'going underground,' that is, becoming submerged again in deep ecology. Secondly, the time frames we deal with are often too short, and I'm sure that there are many microbes that may evolve but quickly disappear, and we would be unlikely to notice these extinctions unless we are either lucky or something calls the organism to our attention, like a disease outbreak."

Viral extinctions have probably occurred repeatedly throughout history. "Possible examples are Rocio encephalitis in Brazil and o'nyong-nyong in Africa," said Morse. "Both appeared in sudden outbreaks and then disappeared. Extinction has been, or can be, invoked for some of the 'mysterious' diseases of the past which defy identification by infections known today, for example the 'sweating sickness' or 'Picardy sweats' in England in 1485, and recurring several times until 1551, and some of the plagues of antiquity."

Certain strains of influenza viruses, because of their propensity for fast mutation, have probably become extinct as well. "Influenza is not only evolving, it is disappearing," said Robert G. Webster, an influenza specialist. "H7 influenza viruses haven't been seen clinically in the world for the last ten years. We did a survey and we can find some evidence in Outer Mongolia and Poland, but otherwise this particular strain of the flu has disappeared."

Even the fabled Marburg virus might conceivably have gone the way of all flesh. It last appeared in western Kenya in 1989, had not been seen since, and there was no guarantee that it would ever turn up again, anywhere in the world. There was a finite number of viruses out there in nature, and there was every reason to think that the total number was decreasing—especially if there were no "new" ones waiting in the wings.

"I personally doubt that there are many left," said Karl M. Johnson, former chief of the CDC's Special Pathogens Branch. "We have hacked and slashed our way into just about all of the unique ecologic niches on the globe. Perhaps ironically, the year 1976, taken by some as the emergence year of modern biotechnology, is also the year that marks the emergence of the last new hemorrhagic fever," Ebola.

Ebola, unfortunately, did not conveniently pass from the scene following the Kikwit crisis. In November 1995 a single new case appeared when a twenty-five-year-old Liberian by the name of Jasper Chea came to a medical clinic in the Ivory Coast with high fever and bloody diarrhea, signs that the doctors quickly sized up as a possible case of Ebola fever. They put him in quarantine, took a blood sample, and sent it off to the Pasteur Institute in Paris, where Bernard Le Guenno found that it indeed carried Ebola antibodies.

Jasper Chea, however, recovered completely.

Two months later, toward the end of January 1996, Ebola broke out in Gabon, in the remote village of Mayibout on the river Ivindo, after a couple of children stumbled upon a dead chimpanzee. Chimpanzees were a delicacy in the region and there was an immediate village feast, the townspeople skinning the animal and cutting it up. But the chimp was harboring the Ebola virus and on January 28, two days after the feast, eighteen cases of Ebola hemorrhagic fever appeared simultaneously in Mayibout.

Bernard Le Guenno now flew to Libreville, took a plane to the town of Makokou in the interior of the country, and boarded a motorized pirogue for a seven-hour cruise up the Ivindo to the village.

In Mayibout, a settlement of about two hundred, the hospital consisted of a few tents. By the time Le Guenno arrived there most of the patients had been transferred to a bigger facility in Makokou, but he and Gabonese public health workers quarantined new cases and put a stop to further transmission, and in the end there would be only about twenty-five cases, and twelve deaths, due to Ebola infection.

And then, finally, Ebola paid a repeat visit to the United States. It had entered the country the first time in 1989, when it caused the original Reston outbreak plus a parallel outbreak in a colony of research monkeys in Philadelphia. In 1990 there was a second Ebola outbreak at the Reston monkey house, and a similar one at the Texas Primate Center, about fifteen miles southeast of Alice, Texas, where forty-four monkeys died of the Ebola Reston virus and another one hundred were destroyed as a precaution.

In none of those cases had there been any human casualties, and so in April 1996, when a monkey newly imported from the Philippines developed signs of hemorrhagic fever and then died at the Texas Primate Center, there was no cause for panic, even after USAMRIID, who'd done the work in the original Reston case, found Ebola particles in liver sections taken from the animal, and the CDC confirmed the results. By this time, Ebola Reston was regarded as posing no special threat to human beings.

"It appears to be of little or no virulence for humans," said CDC lab chief Tom Ksiazek of the virus. "But it's a very bad disease for monkeys."

Still, out of a total population of five thousand monkeys at the Texas Primate Center, only one died of Ebola. A second monkey became sick, was killed, and was found to contain the Ebola virus. Forty-eight other monkeys in the same room were then killed and examined, but only one harbored the virus. That was the total extent of the outbreak; the other 4,950 monkeys remained alive and healthy, and there was no infection among human workers at the facility.

The CDC, nevertheless, sent Pierre Rollin and two others to Alice, Texas, to investigate the incident, and sent Tom Ksiazek, Ali Khan, Anthony Sanchez, and veterinarian Charles Fulhorst to the Philippines, where the diseased monkeys had come from. All told, the CDC scientists and local public health workers would take several thousand blood samples from caged monkeys and their human caretakers.

The outside world remained unnaturally calm in the face of all this, and for the first time in the golden age of virus paranoia there was no talk of Ebola's latest fleeting appearance as portending "the end of civilization." Even Bill Clinton, who just a year earlier had spoken of Ebola as threatening "an entire continent," was unusually restrained when, in an April 15 news conference, he spoke about the Texas event.

"We believe, based on what we now know, that there is no substantial threat to the general population of the people there, or of the people of the United States generally. I would urge people not to overreact to this. It's a serious matter, we are on top of it. I'm confident that the federal government is taking appropriate action and that we're on top of it and there is nothing for people to overreact to at this moment."

The CDC, after all, was on the scene. The disease cowboys had arrived. The Texas Rangers of public health were riding through the viral outback, hot on the trail of masked microbes.

Acknowledgments

This book was researched in Atlanta, Georgia; Frederick, Maryland; Eastham, Massachusetts; and in Brussels, Paris, Geneva, Kinshasa, and Kikwit. In Kinshasa I am indebted to Erik Jacobs for arranging flawless arrival and departure protocols at Aéroport de N'Djili, and to pilot Yves Nisot (who was born in Bumba and who, as a child, often swam in the Ebola River) for a fabulous flight to Kikwit. In Kikwit, special thanks to Manuela Cardoso, former president of La Croix Rouge de Kikwit.

My work was supported in part by a research grant from the Alfred P. Sloan Foundation. I am indebted to the officers of the Foundation, particularly Raphael Kasper, for their assistance.

For clippings, sources, contacts, advice, or other help, I wish to thank W. Emmet Barkley, Ian Bray, William T. Close, Erin Dingle, Laurie Garrett, Robin Henig, Joe Jones, Graham Messick, Fitzhugh Mullan, Jean Naggar, John Parascandola, Doris Regis, Frank Thompson, Paul Tumey, Bill Watson, and Claire Zion. Thanks to Elizabeth Etheridge, author of *Sentinel for Health: A History of the Centers for Disease Control*, for important aid at several points. Special thanks to Roger and Char Musser for research help and a variety of favors, and to FedEx courier Rich DeMartino, who on two occasions during the blizzard of 1996 hiked half a mile through ice and snow to deliver documents.

Several people concerned with the Kikwit episode went out of their way to provide slides, prints, videotapes, medical records, personal documents, or to offer detailed accounts of their participation: Simon Van Nieuwenhove (Belgian Development Cooperation, Brussels), David Heymann and Mark Szczeniowski (WHO, Geneva), Bernard Le Guenno (Pasteur Institute, Paris), and Joanna Buffington (CDC, Atlanta). Thanks to Peter Jahrling (USAMRIID, Frederick, Maryland) for a private tutorial on the ELISA test.

For reading and checking one or more portions of the manuscript, I am indebted to Anthony Sanchez (CDC) and to Stephen S. Morse (Rockefeller University), neither of whom are responsible for any errors that remain, or for the views, interpretations, or conclusions expressed herein. For tape transcription, many thanks to Virginia Story and Pat Holford, and to Colette M. Henriette for translations from the French.

My two editors at Pocket Books, Claire Zion and Julie Rubenstein, offered comments and suggestions that materially improved the text, and for this, many thanks. I owe a special debt to my wife, Pamela Regis, for convincing me that I could complete the project within a demanding time frame, and for her constant help during the course of it. I am most deeply obligated to my literary agent, Jean V. Naggar, for her calming influence, sound advice, and for performing several miracles on my behalf.

Two people who appear early in the narrative are identified by pseudonyms: Loki M'Bele, Claudia.